From its deep roots in the earliest Christian traditions, Patricia Gabow traces the rise of the American Catholic hospital and its transformation into one of the most powerful forces shaping healthcare and health policy today. Her book helps readers of all faiths more fully understand the healthcare and equity challenges we face today, especially when it comes to reproductive health. Dr. Gabow's stature as one of the nation's leading figures in healthcare, and her deep commitment to the Church's original healing mission, give her recommendations for greater health equity even more power.

Sara Rosenbaum, JD
Professor Emerita, Health Law and Policy
Milken Institute School of Public Health
George Washington University

Dr. Gabow's vocation for over 50 years, serving as a Catholic physician, researcher, and patient advocate, especially for the poor and most vulnerable patients, informs her insightful reflection on Catholic healthcare in the United States. Affirming its historical roots, grounded in Jesus' compassion and healing ministry and incarnated through the unwavering commitment of nuns and religious orders, she provides critical insight into the current organizational and operational structures of Catholic healthcare. She proposes ways to move forward by returning to the original mandate of Catholic healthcare grounded in the Gospel and more fully committed to Catholic social teaching.

Todd Salzman, PhD
Amelia and Emil Graff Professor of Catholic Theology
Department of Theology
Creighton University

What enables a group of less than 300 Catholic bishops to define the healthcare of millions of Americans — 80% who are not Catholic? Why don't patients know – often until it's too late – that Catholic healthcare systems are prohibited from performing certain procedures? Why are the bishops not enforcing the foundational Catholic healthcare mission of serving the poor and vulnerable, as Catholic health systems often fail to provide a fair share of community benefits in exchange for their non-profit tax exemptions?

Dr. Patricia A. Gabow is asking all the right questions in this penetrating examination of how Catholic hospitals in the United States have transformed from humble facilities founded by orders of sisters with a mission to serve the poor into giant multi-state healthcare corporations with billions of dollars in assets that are governed by religious doctrine handed down by the US Conference of Catholic Bishops. Dr. Gabow is well-positioned to ask these questions, as a national leader in care of vulnerable populations during her 20 years as CEO of Denver Health, a safety-net hospital system, in her role as Chair of the Board of the Lown Institute and, perhaps most importantly, as a practicing Catholic who is dismayed that Catholic hospitals have "lost their way."

We can pray that her suggestions for needed reforms find sympathetic ears at the Vatican and among public policymakers in the US who must do more to protect patients from denials of basic healthcare at Catholic hospitals that receive tax dollars and may be the only healthcare option for patients in large geographic regions of our country.

Lois J. Uttley, MPP
Health Policy and Advocacy Consultant
Faculty Member, Master's in Health Advocacy Program
Sarah Lawrence College

An inspiring critique of Catholic healthcare today, made even more powerful by the author's obvious love and respect for her church, its belief systems, and its remarkable history in healthcare. When Dr. Gabow asks why Catholic social teachings about care for the poor have become mere recommendations, while its restrictions around sex and reproductive care have become iron-clad rules, the reader feels her visceral frustration. And lest you think this book is only for Catholics, the arguments she lays out apply in equal or greater measure to state laws that implement similar restrictions on medical care, using the power of the state to enforce religious edicts.

Matthew Wynia, MD, MPH
Director, Center for Bioethics and Humanities
Professor, School of Medicine and Colorado School of Public Health
University of Colorado, Anschutz Medical Campus

The Catholic Church and Its Hospitals: A Marriage Made in Heaven?

Patricia A. Gabow, MD, MACP

Foreword by Donald M. Berwick, MD, MPP

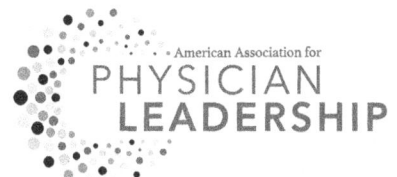

Copyright © 2023 by **American Association for Physician Leadership®**
978-1-960762-09-2 Paperback
978-1-960762-10-8 eBook

Published by **American Association for Physician Leadership, Inc.**
PO Box 96503 | BMB 97493 | Washington, DC 20090-6503

Website: www.physicianleaders.org

All rights reserved. No part of this publication may be reproduced, stored in a retrieval system, or transmitted in any form or by any means, electronic, mechanical, photocopying, recording or otherwise, without prior written permission of the American Association for Physician Leadership. Routine photocopying or electronic distribution to others is a copyright violation.

AAPL books are available at special quantity discounts to use as premiums and sales promotions, or for use in corporate training programs. For more information, please write to Special Sales at journal@physicianleaders.org

This publication is designed to provide general information and is sold with the understanding that neither the author nor the publisher is engaged in rendering legal, accounting, ethical, or clinical advice. If legal or other expert advice is required, the services of a competent professional person should be sought.

13   8 7 6 5 4 3 2 1

Copyedited, typeset, indexed, and printed in the United States of America

PUBLISHER
Nancy Collins

PRODUCTION MANAGER
Jennifer Weiss

DESIGN & LAYOUT
Carter Publishing Studio

COPYEDITOR
Pat George

To the thousands of women religious who courageously and authentically followed the example of Jesus, reaching out to the vulnerable and the sick with compassion and mercy, creating places of caring and healing. May their spirit and example continue to guide Catholic healthcare in America.

ACKNOWLEDGMENTS

This book would not have been possible without a generous gift from Merle Chambers who believed this project was worthy of her support. I had the privilege of working with Nancy Collins at American Association for Physician Leadership who embraced the book's concept and offered valuable advice throughout the process.

I am grateful to Evon Holladay, MBA, who ferreted out information from the health system's financial reports and IRS 990 forms. I owe thanks to the individuals who responded to my queries with helpful information, including:

- Patrick Kampert (Providence St. Joseph Health)
- Adrienne Webb (SSM Health)
- Kathleen Quinn-Leering (ACGME)
- Susan White Holub (ACGME)
- John Coombes (ACGME)
- Jack Resnick, Jr, MD (AMA)
- David Uebbing (Archdiocese of Denver)
- Tari Hanneman (Human Rights Campaign Foundation)
- Kush Banerjee (The Leapfrog Group)
- Elizabeth Griffin (Catholic Medical Association)
- Vikas Saini, MD (Lown Institute)
- Carissa Fu (Lown Institute)
- Judith Garber (Lown Institute).

I am grateful to the archivists who provided material and the images for the book, including Mary Catherine Kzusko (Franciscan Media), Carolyn Ferguson (Seton Shrine), Scott Keefer (Daughters of Charity, Province of St. Louis), Veronica Buchanan (Sisters of Charity of Cincinnati), JoAnn Seaman (Mother Cabrini Shrine), Scott Grimwood (Franciscan Sisters of Mary), Peter Schmid (Providence Archives), and Tonya Crawford (Sisters of Charity of Leavenworth).

I am indebted to my friends and colleagues who read the drafts and provided encouragement, valuable insights, and suggestions, including Michael Baxter, PhD; Tomas Berl, MD; Sharon Caulfield, JD; Michael Earnest, MD; Vicki Earnest, MSN; Darlene Ebert, JD; Lee Ebert; Father Daniel Leonard; Lynne Neefe, MD; Abraham Nussbaum, MD; Diane Pincus, MD; and Stephanie Thomas, MBA.

Finally, I thank my family. My daughter and son encouraged me throughout my work on this project. My husband, Hal, for 52 years has supported me in everything I have ever done. He read the entire manuscript and offered both small changes, challenging questions, valuable insights, and the entire range of computer support.

CONTENTS

Acknowledgments	viii
About the Author	xiii
Foreword	xv
Donald M. Berwick, MD, MPP	
Introduction	1

Chapter 1: The Foundations of Healing   7

    The Value of a Human Being   7
    Healings in the Old Testament   9
    Healings in the New Testament   10
    Healing Given Freely to All   13
    Linking the Care of the Sick with Catholic Institutions   14
    The First Hospital   16
    Conclusion   16

Chapter 2: The Beginnings of Catholic Healthcare in America   19

    Responding to the Call for Help   22
    Catholic Hospitals and Black Americans   25
    Enabling the Care   29
    Catholic Hospitals and Community Physicians   30
    Nuns in a Man's World   32
    Conclusion   33

Chapter 3: Exemplary Mothers   35

    Mother Marianne Cope   35
    Mother Francis Cabrini   37
    Mother Joseph   40
    Mother Odilia Berger   42
    Mother Elizabeth Seton   45
    Conclusion   48

Chapter 4: The Hierarchy and the Rules   49

    The Hierarchy   49
    The Laity   55
    The Rules   56
        Evolution of Ethical and Religious Directives for Catholic Health Care Services (ERDs)   56

    An Elucidation of the Sixth Edition of the ERDs 60
    Conclusion of and Reactions to the Directives 68
    The Good Samaritan (Samaritanus Bonus) End-of-Life Care 69
Conclusion 70

Chapter 5: The Impact of the Rules on Patient Care 73

    Catholic Healthcare's Reach 73
    Contraception 80
        Emergency Contraception 85
    Abortion 85
    Complications of Pregnancy 88
    Infertility 90
    Genetic Disorders 91
    LGBTQ+ Care 92
    End-of-Life Care 95
    Transparency 98
    Conclusion 102

Chapter 6: Fulfilling Oaths and Following Conscience 103

    Impact on Physicians 103
        Trainees 103
        Physicians 104
    Catholic Healthcare, ERDs, and the Law 109
    Conclusion 115

Chapter 7: The Landscape of Catholic Healthcare 117

    Financial Forces 117
    Non-financial Forces 121
    Becoming Corporate 122
        Intermountain Health 124
        CommonSpirit Health 128
        Providence St. Joseph Health Care 131
        Ascension Health 132
        Trinity Health 133
        Bon Secours Mercy Health 135
        SSM Health 135
    A Bump in the Financial Road 137
    Conclusion 137

Chapter 8: Mission Fidelity — 139
Mission Statements   139
Care for the Poor and Vulnerable   140
Community Benefit   146
Financial Profiles   149
Executives vs Employees   153
Patient Care   156
Conclusion   157

Chapter 9: Walking the Old Path and Building New Roads — 159
The Church and Change   160
  The Hierarchy   161
  Women Religious Congregations   165
  The Body of the Church   165
Government   166
  Rules of Conscience   166
  Tax Exemptions   168
Professional Organizations   169
Conclusion   170

References — 171

ABOUT THE AUTHOR

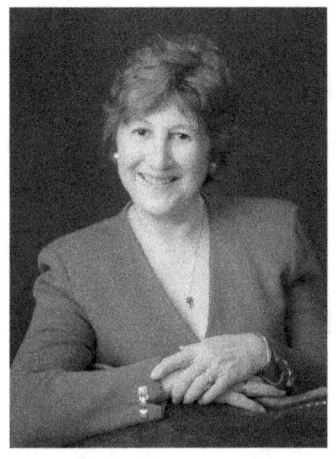

Patricia A. Gabow, MD, is a national healthcare leader who has focused on the care of vulnerable populations and the institutions that serve them. She spent 40 years at Denver Health, a highly integrated healthcare system and Colorado's major safety net institution. The last 20 of those years was as CEO, retiring in 2012.

She began her career as an academic clinician and researcher in the area of renal disease. Dr. Gabow's healthcare leadership career led from head of the renal service to director of the medical services (chair) to the system's medical director to CEO. While CEO she transformed a struggling public hospital system into a model integrated, high-quality, fiscally stable system.

As a healthcare and health policy leader, Dr. Gabow has served on the Commonwealth Commission on a High Performing Health System, the federal Medicaid and CHIP Payment and Access Commission (MACPAC), is currently on the Robert Wood Johnson Foundation Board (2013–2024) and chairs the Lown Institute Board.

She has authored over 130 articles, 36 book chapters, and two books, including *The Lean Prescription: Powerful Medicine for Our Ailing Healthcare System* and *TIME'S NOW for Women Healthcare Leaders: A Guide for the Journey*.

Dr. Gabow's numerous awards include the American Medical Association Nathan Davis Award for Outstanding Public Service, the Association of Medical College's David E. Rogers Award, the Health Quality Leader Award from the National Committee for Quality Assurance, The National Healthcare Leadership Award, the Gustav O. Lienhard Award from the National Academy of Medicine, and the Ohtli Award from the Mexican government.

She was elected to the Association for Manufacturing Hall of Fame and the National Academy for Social Insurance. Dr. Gabow has received honorary degrees from the University of Colorado School of Medicine and the University of Denver.

She graduated from Seton Hill University and the Perlman School of Medicine of the University of Pennsylvania. She is Professor Emerita of the University of Colorado School of Medicine and a Master of the American College of Physicians.

FOREWORD

Donald M. Berwick, MD, MPP
*President Emeritus and Senior Fellow,
Institute for Healthcare Improvement*

Speaking truth to power is not for wimps — even less so when the power is palatial and the truth is a threat to its incumbency. Dr. Patricia Gabow is not now, nor has she in my experience ever been, daunted by the risks of truth-telling. This book testified to her courage.

For the decades of her leadership as CEO of Denver Health, an admired and successful integrated safety net care system, and for a decade since as a continuing presence on the landscape of American healthcare, Dr. Gabow has vocally championed the interests of the far-too-many excluded, underserved, and marginalized people in our nation.

She has unblinkingly forced attention to failures in policy and finance to bring resources to the people who need them most. She has called for and modeled the leadership of women in the male-dominated corporate healthcare industry. She has argued for bold strengthening of Medicaid and other components of the safety net, and she has called out hypocritical behaviors and avarice in healthcare where she has seen them. She has been unafraid to ring alarms even in the inner sanctums of the highest executive levels in the healthcare industry, where the more customary social norms more often eschew self-criticism or even honest interrogation of the data.

To be clear, the data on the performance of American healthcare are not reassuring. It is true – and no less true because it is now so often repeated – that the U.S. healthcare system costs per capita nearly twice that of the next most expensive nation on earth, and that summative metrics of American health – such as infant mortality, life expectancy, and racial and class inequities in health status – show shortfalls that are more flagrant by far than any other western developed nation.

Our investments in the "repair shops" that American hospitals are reach orders of magnitude greater than in the prevention and social supports that, we know from data and science, reduce the need for repair – and save money.

American healthcare costs are an embarrassment. Prices of healthcare products and services in the U.S. water the eyes of European observers, who simply cannot believe that we spend so much to obtain what they can get for a fraction of what we pay. Medical debt, which today encumbers 110 million Americans, is nearly unknown in other wealthy nations. And universal health insurance – guaranteed one way another to every person – has been achieved in every single wealthy nation on earth except one: the USA. In failing to guarantee healthcare as a human right, we are starkly, astonishingly, immorally, alone.

Dr. Gabow has directed her entire career in large measure to setting these things right. In this, she has earned the respect and gratitude of clinicians, executives, policymakers, and philanthropists throughout the U.S., and, indeed, abroad. Now, in this book, she directs her spotlight and intelligence to a matter edgier than almost anything she has reported on before: the activities of Catholic healthcare, for better and, substantially, for worse.

She is no neutral party in this expedition. Throughout this book, Dr. Gabow lets her Catholic roots and persisting affection for the Church shine clearly. She devotes chapters to the earliest teaching of the religion, and to those of Jesus in the Gospels, which she honors. Her accounts preclude surprise that the Church, heeding its own deepest teachings, eventually found its way into sponsorship of hospitals and other healthcare organizations.

She reserves glowing praise for the many "women religious," nuns, some eventually canonized, who founded the original hospitals in the U.S. that today have morphed and grown into some of the nation's largest multi-hospital systems, such as Common Spirit, Ascension, Providence, SSM, Bon Secours Mercy, and Trinity. In much of the history that Dr. Gabow reports in scholarly detail, the genetic line connecting the charity and compassion espoused in the Gospels and the founding of Catholic hospitals is clear and credible.

But something goes wrong. Without drama or exaggeration, Dr. Gabow describes the reshaping of Catholic healthcare more and more by financial forces, mergers and acquisitions, business strategies, and corporate ambition. She presents data showing, if not the erosion of the charitable mission of the founding women religious, then at least the admixture of corporate behaviors that are hard to reconcile with the words of the Gospels or, frankly, with the mission statements of the large hospital systems, themselves.

Catholic healthcare systems are as likely as other healthcare systems – for-profit and not-for-profit – to pursue debt collection from patients who have difficulty paying, to amass enormous amounts of money on their balance sheets, to trim investments in community benefit, and to pay executives handsomely. Dr. Gabow reports that the compensation packages of the five highest paid executives at Ascension health would cover the salaries of 331 registered nurses or 903 healthcare housekeepers. For Common Spirit, the numbers are 301 nurses or 821 housekeepers.

She cites independent rankings of 296 hospital systems for investments in community benefit, for example, which show Catholic systems far from a leadership position: Ascension ranks 134, Bon Secours Mercy ranks 165, and Providence 158.

Scholars studying the ways in which American healthcare falls short of its promise will recognize that the Catholic systems are not exceptional in the degree of that gap. But the gap seems especially egregious when compared with the rhetoric of mission and charitable intent that every Catholic system espouses, and even more when compared to the words of Catholic philosophers and clerics through the ages. From the Gospel of Matthew: *"Cure the sick...cleanse the lepers...Without cost you have received; without cost you are to give."* Dr. Gabow quotes Abraham Lincoln who said, after visiting a hospital staffed by nuns: *"Of all the forms of charity and benevolence seen in the crowded wards of the hospitals, those of the Catholic Sisters were among the most efficient."* After reading Dr. Gabow's updated history, one thinks, "Today, not so much."

In a parallel excavation of the behaviors of Catholic healthcare, Dr. Gabow explains the central role of the "Ethical and Religious Directives for Catholic Health Care Services" (ERDs) issued by the United States Congress of Catholic Bishops about 75 years ago and revised at least five times since. The ERDs instruct Catholic hospitals and the clinicians within them about what they may and may not do in their care according to Church law.

The directives – some 77 in all – cover a wide range of clinical and organizational behaviors, and many contain specific instructions on patient care. Abortion, birth control, and assisted suicide are prohibited, for example, and a physician in a Catholic system may not refer patients to other systems for such care.

Dr. Gabow takes these ERDs as part of the political and doctrinal landscape at least for now (though she would change many of them), but she hastens to point out that many of the patients cared for in Catholic hospitals are not Catholic, and that, in essence, the Church through the ERDs is molding their care as well, and often without transparency. She calls into question this imperial extension of power and argues for far more transparency.

She notes that few of the websites of Catholic systems make their Catholic affiliations easily visible, and almost none advise readers that, if they become patients, they will be subjected to the ERD restrictions, whether they are Catholic or not.

As she walks the reader from the origins of Catholic healthcare through its growth and into the modern, troubled, and ambivalent, if not outright hypocritical, era, Dr. Gabow maintains a voice that manages to be at once deeply respectful and verging on outrage.

She offers specific suggestions for reform and the reestablishment of the healing mission in truth at the center of Catholic healthcare, and she almost pleads with the incumbent power – largely men and many aged – to interrogate their rules and behaviors against the root teaching of the Church.

What I find most remarkable about this brief for authentic reform is not its intelligence, clarity, and documentary scholarship. These are traits Dr. Gabow has long exhibited to those of us fortunate enough to know her.

Most remarkable to me is the realization that this is, after all, a love story. Dr. Gabow loves the Church, try though she may sometimes to hide that. But it is the story also, of love spurned – disappointed – as Dr. Gabow shows the distance between what Catholic healthcare claims to be and could be, on the one hand – guided by compassion, generosity, healing, and justice above all – and what it has, too much, become – controlled by finance, seeking growth and power, and unwisely testing the boundaries between its ethical heritage and the imperatives of today's market-driven myths.

Will Dr. Gabow's truth-to-power adventure yield change? One can only hope.

INTRODUCTION

Catholic healthcare occupies a large and growing footprint in American healthcare, and across the American landscape with facilities cropping up in farm country and emerging in urban centers. The vast system of Catholic healthcare we see today is actually quite surprising. In the first half of the 1800s, only 5% of Americans were Catholic and although that number grew to 13% by 1900, much of that growth was due to the arrival of mostly poor immigrants.

One powerful driving force enabled this growth of the Catholic healthcare system: the Catholic women religious — the nuns — coming from Europe, who were tirelessly and fearlessly committed to living Jesus' example of healing all who came to him. Catholic healthcare had a humble beginning. The nuns established small hospitals in the teeming cities and the remote territories of the Wild West to serve those in need.

Today, those hospitals have evolved into multi-billion-dollar healthcare corporations comprised of hospitals, physician groups, outpatient facilities, insurance companies, and even venture capital companies. Four of the 10 largest U.S. healthcare systems, in monetary terms, are Catholic systems. In some states, more than 40% of the hospital beds are in Catholic hospitals. One of the largest Catholic systems, CommonSpirit, claims that one in four Americans have access to healthcare in its system.

Reflecting this reach, Catholic hospitals deliver large volumes of healthcare to the American people. For example, in 2020 almost 500,000 babies — 15% of all the babies born in the United States — entered the world in a Catholic hospital. Added to those numbers of deliveries are millions of clinic and emergency department visits and hospital stays.

If the magnitude of care provided by Catholic healthcare were the entire story, there would be nothing to do but offer gratitude. There would be no questions to ask, no concerns to raise. But it is not that simple.

These hospitals and the many other components of the healthcare systems owned by Catholic systems, and some with whom they are affiliated, function under the supervision of the Catholic bishops. These entities must comply with 77 rules known as the Ethical and Religious Directives for Catholic Health Care Services (ERDs). The ERDs were first published in 1948 and have been reissued multiple times, most recently in 2018.

Beyond the prohibition of abortion, neither the scope of the rules nor their implications for care are well-known to patients, to communities, or even to those with their finger on the healthcare pulse. The ERDs cover a large swath of healthcare, from commitment to social responsibility including care of the poor, to spiritual care, to the definitions of the beginning and end of life and the attendant prohibitions of some care and procedures, to relationships and mergers with other entities.

Part of the lack of knowledge about the rules that govern Catholic healthcare stems from the fact that there is little transparency about the Catholic ownership of a given hospital and a hospital's enforcement of the ERDs, including the wide range of prohibited care. Patients believe that their care will be determined solely by standards of medical care and what the physician believes to be in their best interest. They often are unaware that the physicians who care for them in Catholic hospitals, emergency departments, and clinics must obey all the prohibitions within the ERDs.

The myriad prohibitions in care lead to the question, "What enables a group of less than 300 Catholic bishops to define the healthcare of millions of Americans, 80% of whom are not Catholic?"

This is really a two-part question. The first part of the question focuses on the power of the American bishops. The hierarchical structure of the Catholic Church establishes the bishops' ability to oversee and direct practices of Catholic institutions, even ones they do not directly operate or fund.

The second part of the question focuses on how this power can extend beyond the members of the Catholic Church. The answer to this begins with the First Amendment of the Constitution and free exercise of religion. This freedom has been amplified by a subsequent series of so called "conscience laws" which give individual healthcare providers and healthcare organizations the right to exercise their own beliefs, even when those beliefs may not comport to those of the patients for whom they are caring.

Compliance with the rules of a single religious group in the delivery of healthcare, which is funded primarily with public dollars and advantaged by tax-exemptions, gives rise to many implications and issues for patients, for a community, and for the entire healthcare system in our pluralistic country. Therefore, this entire terrain deserves broad and meaningful exploration.

Although there is a body of literature on Catholic healthcare, it is often presented from a single perspective, frequently its history or its theology.

However, there are many relevant perspectives from which to view and, most importantly, to measure Catholic healthcare in America: theological, historical, mission-centric, patient and community, business, and public policy perspectives. All of these are valid, important, and necessary lenses through which to examine this large component of our healthcare system.

The goal of this book is to present information in these areas to a wide audience of government officials, policy makers, healthcare leaders, physicians, advocates, and all of us who use healthcare, in order to generate an understanding of this system, expand the dialogue about the provision of Catholic healthcare, and going forward, to build on what is good and explore what should be changed.

The chapters are organized to flow across time from the Biblical age to the present day and across perspectives from the theological to public policy, detailing the evolution of Catholic healthcare from its roots to its current structure. The theological perspectives embedded in the Old and New Testaments are worth understanding as they give rise to the Church's commitment to healing from its earliest days (Chapter 1).

A foundational tenet is the intrinsic value, worth, and uniqueness of a human being. This simple tenet is the foundation of many principles applied to Catholic healthcare. Jesus' teaching and, more importantly, his life are the cornerstones of Catholicism and Catholic healthcare. His example of healing those in need out of mercy and compassion and his inclusion of all, especially those on the margins of society, became the path for healthcare to follow.

The intent of Chapter 1 is not to debate the spiritual, moral, or religious validity of any beliefs, but rather to simply present them. The early history of Christianity is also laid out in Chapter 1 as it is useful in providing an understanding of how the Church, the hospital, and healthcare became tightly linked.

American healthcare was built by thousands of nuns operationalizing that commitment to healing, especially of the poor (Chapters 2 and 3). Their stories of unwavering zeal in overcoming hardship and their willingness to put their own lives at risk to care for those abandoned by others serve as both an inspiration and a template with which to view Catholic healthcare today.

The straightforward work of caring for those in need in those first Catholic hospitals in America changed as the science of medicine advanced, forces shaping healthcare delivery emerged, and society and Catholic leadership changed. The ERDs were a response/reaction to that evolution.

The goals of ERDs are to link Catholic teachings and beliefs to relevant aspects of healthcare delivery, to ensure conformity to Catholic beliefs across all Catholic healthcare, and to formalize the bishops' supervisory roles (Chapter 4). The ERDs and other communications from Popes and bishops are detailed to enable a grasp of the basis and scope of the rules that govern Catholic healthcare in America.

The ERDs and other Church rules have numerous important healthcare implications for patients, especially related to procreation, sexuality, and end-of-life care. Given the breadth of prohibited care, it is concerning that there is lack of transparency about this from the healthcare institutions. Since these institutions exist for the primary purpose of providing healthcare, patients expect this care to be delivered and should be informed if it will not be given (Chapter 5). The interaction of the ERDs, the physicians' professional oath and duties of care, and the exercise of providers' and institutions' religious beliefs can create dilemmas for physicians as well as patients (Chapter 6).

Over the last half century many financial and non-financial forces have altered American healthcare, including Catholic healthcare. Those forces transformed Catholic hospitals from small organizations run by nuns to large healthcare systems. These organizations now have lay leaders and are highly profitable business entities (Chapter 7). This seismic transformation raises the question, "Do these vast, complex Catholic healthcare systems have fidelity to their theological and historical missions?" (Chapter 8).

This winding journey of the evolution of Catholic healthcare cannot end with only dilemmas and questions. Therefore, the concluding chapter (Chapter 9) provides some possible paths forward for Catholic healthcare to respond to known and emerging medical knowledge, to a broad range of voices in the Church, to have mission fidelity, and to function more openly and fairly in a pluralistic nation.

I approach this discussion as a physician and healthcare leader for many decades, and as a life-long practicing Catholic. I was raised in an Italian Catholic family, being put to bed as a young child with the stories of the saints, and as a high school student, discussing with my uncle books by Catholic thinkers like G.K. Chesterton. I attended a Catholic university being personally mentored by the Sisters of Charity. I have valued Catholic thinkers and Catholic Social Teaching and embraced the Catholic faith.

I believe all of this contributed to my becoming a physician and choosing to practice in a safety-net healthcare system.

I have been fortunate to have had many diverse opportunities to participate in our healthcare system: being an academic physician caring for patients for more than 50 years; leading a large safety-net healthcare system committed to the care of the poorest and most vulnerable for 20 years; engaging in research to improve care and reform the system; and participating in health policy through governmental and philanthropic organizations for decades.

Each of these lived experiences created different perspectives and important learnings. Caring for poor patients revealed the difficult realities they face beyond their illness. Working in a safety-net healthcare system revealed the barriers that are often erected to those most in need, even by Catholic healthcare institutions. It underscored the importance of an institutional commitment in removing those barriers. Research demonstrated the value of science and the importance of applying new knowledge in caring for patients. Interactions with policy makers and government leaders revealed their importance in shaping and overseeing our healthcare system.

These multiple experiences led me to ask the following questions about Catholic healthcare, to try to answer these questions, and finally to write this book:

- Are healing and healthcare linked to the bedrock foundations of Catholicism?
- Why and how did Catholic healthcare become established in America?
- What role have the Catholic hierarchy and Catholic beliefs had in shaping American healthcare?
- How do Catholic beliefs and rules affect patient care and physicians who care for these patients?
- Are Catholic hospitals and healthcare entities transparent about the rules they follow and how that affects patients?
- What enables the Catholic Church to direct the healthcare of millions of Americans, most of whom are not Catholic?
- Does Catholic healthcare, as currently practiced, authentically reflect its foundations and Catholic Social Teaching?
- What are the questions posed for public policy by Catholic healthcare in America today?
- Are there changes that could and should happen with Catholic healthcare?

This book examines these questions utilizing published literature and articles, through the exploration of current databases, and through individual women's religious orders,' hospitals' and health systems' public-facing information, such as their websites and histories. It does not present every perspective that could be relevant to these questions.

The Catholic Church and Its Hospitals does aim to provide a sufficiently broad and deep perspective on this critical component of American healthcare to stimulate dialogue regarding this system of care — perhaps at the end, answering the question of whether Catholic healthcare was, is, or can truly be a "marriage made in heaven."

CHAPTER 1

The Foundations of Healing

Jesus went around all the towns and villages...proclaiming the gospel...and curing every disease and illness.
                                                    Matthew 9:35

Some readers, especially those who never were or are not currently practicing Jews, Catholics, or Christians, may not be aware of the Biblical, theological, or historical foundations of Catholicism's commitment to healing and care of the sick. However, these concepts create highly relevant context for the story of Catholic healthcare.

Understanding these foundations of healing enables us to evaluate the current system within the framework of Catholicism's essential beliefs. The reader need not embrace the material presented as theological or historical truth. Nonetheless, it is critical to understand the meaning and power of its messages.

Of note, in this chapter, Catholicism is considered identical to early Christianity. Although Catholicism evolved, there was not an abrupt split between Catholicism and Christianity until the Reformation in the 16th century.

THE VALUE OF A HUMAN BEING

Healing and compassion for the sick are inexorably linked to the Judaic-Christian theological concept of what it is to be human. These values and actions are embedded in the origins of human beings as told in Genesis:

"Then God said, 'Let us make human beings in our image, after our likeness'.... God created mankind in his image, in the image of God he created them: male and female he created them. God blessed them.... God looked at everything that he made and found it very good." (Genesis 1: 26,27, 31 The New American Bible Revised Edition, NAB).

If human beings are the image and likeness of God, and if they are very good in God's eyes, they must have infinite value and dignity and, therefore, be worthy of concern and care. This intrinsic worth is a recurring theme in the Old Testament. At least four of the Ten Commandments given by God to Moses dictate a person's relationship and responsibility to others, reflecting this worth:

> *"Honor your father and your mother.... You shall not kill. You shall not bear false witness against your neighbor. You shall not covet your neighbor's ...wife, his male or female slave...." (Exodus 20:12,13,16,17, NAB).*

Psalm 8 in the Old Testament expresses and beautifully sums up the value given to human beings:

> *"... When I see your heavens, the work of your fingers,*
> *the moon and the stars that you set in place—*
> *What is man that you are mindful of him,*
> *and the son of man that you care for him?*
> *Yet you made him little less than a god,*
> *crowned him with glory and honor...." (Psalm 8:4–6 NAB).*

This was a different perspective on the worth of a human being than was the predominant view in the pagan cultures of the time.[1] A powerful reflection of this departure of Judaism from the prevailing culture relates to human sacrifice to the gods. This had no place in the Jewish worship of Yahweh. This prohibition was quite dramatically portrayed in the story in which God asks Abraham to place his son Isaac on an altar and sacrifice him, but then stops Abraham from killing his son, instead providing a ram for sacrifice (Genesis 22 NAB).

Even given this enormous value placed on human life in the Jewish religion of the Old Testament, it was given even greater value in the New Testament by two core and spectacular beliefs:

1. The Incarnation of God in the person of Jesus, who was both fully human and fully divine.
2. That Jesus, both fully divine and fully human, would willingly die for humanity.

While there are stories of pagan gods taking on human forms, they were disguised to deceive. These gods did not intend to imbue humanity with the greatest possible worth nor to bind God and humanity in a sacred relationship. Theirs was a much different relationship.

> *"Whereas the gods of Olympus tirelessly pursued beautiful women, the God of Sinai watched over widows and orphans."*[2]

Pagan gods did not care about the poor nor was caring for the poor seen as part of a relationship with god in pagan societies.[3]

The humanity and divinity of Jesus established a kinship of every person with Jesus and with God. The obligation that emanates from this kinship is to care for every person as if they were Jesus himself. Jesus makes this clear when he indicates who would enter the kingdom of God:

> "For I was hungry and you gave me food, I was thirsty and you gave me drink, ... ill and you cared for me....Then the righteous will answer him and say, 'Lord, when did I see...you ill...And the king will say to them,...whatever you did for one of these least brothers of mine, you did to me." (Matthew 25: 35–40 NAB).

HEALINGS IN THE OLD TESTAMENT

Catholics, and Christians in general, often associate the sending of plagues and other scourges with the Old Testament and miraculous healings with the New Testament. While reports of miraculous healings are fewer in the Old Testament, given the thousands of years encompassed in those texts compared to the short duration of the New Testament period, there are still a substantial number.

In the Old Testament, the healers are primarily Moses and the prophets Elijah and Elisha. Those healed are individuals and the community, the latter often after imposed scourges.

The miracles of Moses are in large part for all Israelites. Foreshadowing the New Testament, Elijah's and Elisha's healings include leprosy, disability, insanity, infertility, and even raising of the dead. Importantly, for understanding the broad commitment to healing and care, and as is reaffirmed in the New Testament, these miracles are not limited to the Jewish people or any specific group. For example, Elisha healed a foreign army commander from leprosy (2 Kings 5:1–14 NAB).

Not only are there miracles for healing, but also for sustaining life. Elijah saves a woman and her son from starvation by causing her meager amount of flour and oil to last for many days (1 Kings 17: 8–16 NAB). Elisha miraculously fills numerous jugs of oil, providing income for a widow and saving her two sons from being sold into slavery (2 Kings 4:1–7 NAB). Elisha multiplies 20 loaves of bread and some grains to provide food for 100 men, even having food remaining (2 Kings 4:42–44 NAB). One of the greatest of these miracles is God feeding the entire migrating tribe of Israelites for 40 years in the desert. It appears the Old Testament is clear about food as one of the social determinants of health!

HEALINGS IN THE NEW TESTAMENT

As a Jew, Jesus came to the synagogue on the Sabbath. In fact, he began his public ministry in the synagogue. There, he read from the writing of the Prophet Isaiah and linked the Old Testament teaching to himself and to his mission to teach and heal:

> *"The Spirit of the Lord is upon me, because he has anointed me to bring glad tidings to the poor. He has sent me to proclaim liberty to captives and recovery of sight to the blind...." (Luke 4:16–19, NAB).*

The New Testament's account of Jesus's life is filled with the miracles he performed. The fact that the majority of the miracles are either healings of specific diseases or conditions in an individual, raising someone from the dead, or supporting human life with food or protection should convey to any reader how central preserving well-being and healing of the body, not just the soul, is to Catholicism. Table 1.1 details these healings: who was healed, what was done, Jesus's motivation, and his teaching in the miracle.

TABLE 1.1. The Physical Healings of Jesus in the New Testament

1. **Who and What:** A man with leprosy who came to Jesus. (Matthew 8:2–4; Mark 1:40–45; Luke 5:12–15) **Why and How:** The leper asked: "Lord, if you will, you can make me clean?" Jesus moved with pity and healed him.
2. **Who and What:** A paralyzed servant of a Roman centurion. (Matthew 8:5–13; Luke 7:1–10) **Why and How:** The centurion begged Jesus to heal the man. Jesus did so because of the centurion's faith.
3. **Who and What:** Peter's mother-in-law with a fever. (Matthew 8:14–15; Mark 1:29–31; Luke 4:38–39) **Why and How:** The disciples told Jesus she was ill and asked him about her; the fever left her.
4. **Who and What:** A paralyzed man brought to Jesus on a bed. (Matthew 9:1–8; Mark 2:1–12; Luke 5:17–26) **Why and How:** His friends lowered him through a roof to get him to Jesus to be healed, which Jesus did.
5. **Who and What:** A woman with hemorrhaging for 12 years. (Matthew 9:20–22; Mark 5:25–34; Luke 8: 43–48) **Why and How:** The woman's faith as she said, "If I only touch his cloak, I shall be cured." Her hemorrhaging stopped immediately.

6. Who and What: Two blind men — one a beggar (Matthew 9:27–31; Mark 10: 46–52; Luke 18:35–43) **Why and How:** The men/man's plea, "Jesus, Son of David, have pity on me." Their sight was restored.
7. Who and What: A man in the synagogue with a withered hand. (Matthew 12: 9–14; Mark 3: 1–6; Luke 6: 6–11). **Why and How:** Jesus was teaching about primacy of mercy and healing over letter of the Law which prohibited work on the Sabbath and healed the withered hand on the Sabbath.
8. Who and What: A blind man. (Mark 8: 22–26) **Why and How:** People brought him to Jesus and asked that he be healed, which Jesus did.
9. Who and What: A woman crippled for 18 years. (Luke 13:10–17) **Why and How:** Jesus simply saw her and healed her, again making a point that it is lawful to heal on the Sabbath.
10. Who and What: A man with dropsy. (Luke 14: 1–6) **Why and How:** The man was "before him"; Jesus healed him, again making a point that it is lawful to heal on the Sabbath.
11. Who and What: Ten lepers came to Jesus. (Luke 17:11–19) **Why and How:** The lepers ask to be healed, "Jesus have pity on us." They were made clean.
12. Who and What: A man ill for 38 years who was lying by a gate in Jerusalem. (John 5: 2–9) **Why and How:** Jesus knew he had been in this state for a long time and asked the man if he wanted to be healed, which he did. The man picked up his mat and walked. It was on the Sabbath.
13. Who and What: A widow's dead son. (Luke 7:11–17) **Why and How:** Jesus saw the funeral procession, had compassion for the widow, and returned the man to his mother alive.
14. Who and What: A dead daughter of Jarius, a synagogue leader. (Matthew 9:18–19,23 25; Mark 5: 21–24,35–43; Luke 8:41–42,49–56). **Why and How:** The father's faith, his saying to Jesus, "Come and lay your hand on her and she will live." And she did.
15. Who and What: Jesus is told his friend Lazarus is dead. (John 11:1–44) **Why and How:** Lazarus' sisters sent a message to Jesus saying, "Master, the one you love is ill." Jesus raised him from the dead.

Adapted from the New American Bible (Revised Edition) 2012

In almost all of the healings, Jesus is responding to a person's need or plea for help. The texts emphasize that he performed the healings to reveal his true nature with its infinite compassion and mercy.[4] One example is the raising of the widow's son from death. As the story is told, Jesus is entering a city and comes upon a funeral procession for the only son of a widow. The widow never speaks or asks for help, but Jesus sees her and knows her great grief.

> "...When the Lord saw her, he was moved with pity for her and said to her, 'Do not weep.' He stepped forward and touched the coffin...and he said, 'Young man, I tell you, arise!' The dead man sat up...and Jesus gave him to his mother." (Luke 7:13–15, NAB)

While there are many healings detailed in the Gospels (Table 1.1), it is worth noting that the Gospel writers clearly conveyed these were only a sampling:

> "Jesus went around all the towns and villages...proclaiming the gospel...and curing every disease and illness." (Matthew 9:35, NAB)

Some healings are characterized as casting out of demons. The nature of these healings cannot be as clearly identified as can the healing of the lepers or the blind. In addition, there are miracles directed at other threats to life and limb, such as feeding thousands of people who came to remote locations to hear Jesus preach (Matthew 14:15–21; Matthew 15: 32–38; Mark 6: 30–44; Mark 8:1–9; Luke 9: 12–17; John 6: 5–13 NAB) and calming dangerous seas (Matthew 14:22–32; Mark 4: 35–39; Mark 6: 45–51; Luke 8: 22–24 NAB).

We can reasonably conclude that there was a clear message in these healings and miracles: As human beings, especially those who profess to follow Jesus, we are to respond to the pleas and needs of others and help them with mercy and compassion and without payment. This is the foundation of Catholicism's commitment to healing.

Jesus reinforces this message with his teachings, particularly in the parable of the Good Samaritan (Luke 10:29–37, NAB). A person trying to understand the directive to love your neighbor as yourself asks Jesus, "*Who is my neighbor?*" Jesus responds with this parable. A Jewish man on a journey is attacked by robbers and left on the roadside. Two men, members of the religious hierarchy, pass him by, but a Samaritan (a group of excluded outsiders) stops and dresses his wounds, takes him to an innkeeper, and pays for his care. After telling the story, Jesus turns the question back to the man, "*Who is the neighbor to the injured man?*" The questioner correctly ascertains, "*The one who showed him mercy.*"

But this lesson does not end with that correct observation. Jesus then says, *"Go and do likewise."* The messages delivered in this story are four-fold:

1. Those who live the principles, and not merely state them, are those who act rightly.
2. It is a human duty to care for others, even others "not in our group."
3. Our caring is using our everyday resources, not miracles.
4. As detailed in the papal document, *Salvifici Doloris,* the suffering of others should give us the reason to act with compassion.[5]

HEALING GIVEN FREELY TO ALL

It is worth examining those with whom Jesus associated, who were the benefactors of Jesus' healings, and what was expected from them in return. He ate with the lower class. He touched the untouchables. Those he healed were either outcasts such as lepers or ones on the margins of that society: the disabled, the poor, the widows, and the beggars (Table 1.1). It was rarely the rich or the powerful.

There seem to be only two powerful persons who benefited from Jesus' healing. A synagogue leader's (Jarius) daughter was raised from the dead. A Roman centurion's servant was healed. Notably, the centurion was a soldier in the occupying army, hardly a friend of the Jewish people. Jesus upended the societal hierarchy of his time; there were no "others," no outcasts, outsiders.[6] Although it was common at that time for anyone who was healed to make a gift to the Temple, Jesus never finished his healings with an ask for a donation, even from those rich men.

Among the reports of Jesus in the New Testament is another message about money. The only time we see Jesus show real anger is when he throws out the merchants and money changers in the Court of the Gentiles in the Temple (Matthew 21:12-14, NAB). People were making money while keeping non-Jews from participating by occupying the area designated for the Gentiles, thereby committing two transgressions — greed and exclusion — transgressions easily committed by any person in power, not only in ancient times but perhaps even more so today.

Many of Jesus' healing miracles enabled the person to return to full function in the community. In this period, just as often in our times, many people with illness or disability, especially those with leprosy, were forced to live outside their communities. Jesus's healing ended the person's isolation — a goal that healthcare should still aspire to.

These miracles and their recounting may have been to convey the divine power of Jesus and to mirror spiritual healing. Still, they also often conveyed the message of how all people should follow the example of Jesus as a human person.[4] It was clearly Jesus' expectation that future Christian leaders continue his teachings and his examples. He directed his Apostles to:

> "Cure the sick...cleanse the lepers.... Without cost you have received; without cost you are to give." (Matthew 10:8, NAB).

The Acts of the Apostles and, to a lesser extent, the Epistles in the New Testament record the continuing commitment to healing the sick. This healing was an important aspect of the new Christian religion. Many historians believe these healings and, even more importantly, the continued commitment to caring activities in the early days of the Church (see below) were major contributors to the rapid rise and spread of Christianity.[1,4,7] This point should not be lost on us today.

LINKING THE CARE OF THE SICK WITH CATHOLIC INSTITUTIONS

Healing was a central component of the ministry of Jesus and the Apostles that could have vanished when they were no longer present. However, it was deeply embedded and sustained in the early centuries following their deaths. In his book *Medicine and Healthcare in Early Christianity*, Ferngren lays out the role of the early Church in the provision of care and its evolution from the first Church communities, in which non-medically trained church leaders and community members cared for their sick members and others in their communities, through the emergence of the hospital.[1]

Notable examples of this caring commitment occurred during the geographically dispersed plagues that hit Europe, the Middle East, and Africa during the early centuries of this era. Not only were the Christians the principal caregivers, but they were also the gravediggers.[1]

In fact, some historians believe that if the plagues in the third and fourth centuries had not occurred and if the Christians had not demonstrated an extraordinary commitment to caring for those not of their faith, often at the expense of their own lives, Christianity would never have moved beyond a small, minor sect.[1,4] Much of the care centered not only around the Christian communities of lay people, but also in the monasteries.

Ferngren points out that the transition to formal hospital care was partly due to Christianity becoming an embraced religion of the Roman Empire in 313 CE.[1] The churches had money to care for the sick and the poor, and when the Church became a mainstream institution, the state came to rely on the Church for its charitable activities. This philanthropy was tax-exempt.[1] (Who knew this construct of the "Grand Bargain" of no taxes in return for community contributions dated back to Constantine?) A prime example of this philanthropy was the hospital:

> *"The hospital was in its origin and conception, a distinctly Christian institution, rooted in the Christian concepts of charity and philanthropy. There were no pre-Christian institutions in the ancient world that served the purpose that the Christian hospitals were created to serve...offering... health care to those in need.... Indeed, in its development and extension of that role lies Christianity's chief contribution to health care."*[1]

The link of Catholicism with healthcare was so foundational that the Council of Nicaea in 325 CE, which was a convening of the hierarchy of the Church and the Empire, required that a hospital be established in every cathedral.[8]

Crislip's book *From the Monastery to Hospital* adds insights into how monastic life created an important perspective regarding those who were ill and an operational approach to the care of the sick within a monastery.[9] The Order of St. Benedict, founded in 529 CE, was the main monastic force in the West. Its Rule specifically focused on care for the sick as a central obligation of the monks:

> *"Before and above all things, care must be taken of the sick, that they be served in very truth as Christ is served; because He hath said: 'I was sick and you visited me (Mt 25:36) And, 'As long as you did to one of these My least brethren, you did it to Me (Mt 25:40).*[10]

Within this monastic philosophy, the sick were not viewed as bringing illness on themselves nor were they ostracized, but rather cared for. In fact, the monasteries may have anticipated by millennia the concept of paid sick leave, as the sick were relieved of many obligations in monastic life.[9]

Given that monastics most often lived completely isolated from the outside world, they needed an organized and structured approach to care for their sick members. Surprisingly, that system included hospital care in a separate unit and ambulatory care in the monk's cell. The care was provided by trained doctors and nurses, some of whom were members of the monastic community.[9] It is not much of a stretch to see how this could have been adapted to society overall, and in fact, it was.

THE FIRST HOSPITAL

The first entity we would recognize as a hospital was probably Basileias in Cappadocia, named for St. Basil, who had visited many monasteries and adapted what he saw to the community.[8] He integrated monastic healthcare, the obligations of bishops to care for the many needs of the poor, and the Eastern knowledge of medicine into the idea of physical buildings staffed by professionals and providing healthcare for rich and poor alike.[8]

The hospital opened in 372 CE. To call it merely a hospital would do it a great injustice as it anticipated by millennia the current efforts of hospitals to go beyond standard medical care to address the broader social determinants of health.

Basileias designated care for six major groups: the poor, strangers and the homeless, orphans, the elderly and infirm, lepers, and those who were ill.[9] The poor, the strangers, and the homeless were housed and fed. The orphans were educated to facilitate their ability to earn a living. The sick were not only treated by trained doctors and nurses, but were prepared to be reintegrated as productive citizens when they were discharged. No one was turned away.

This is astounding by any standards of that time or indeed by our time. No wonder this hospital complex was proclaimed a wonder of the world.[8,9] One could only wish that today's healthcare system, especially the Catholic healthcare system, had as encompassing a mission and was as inclusive as was Basileias.

Other hospitals followed in this part of the country. The first hospital in Europe was probably in 390 CE — where else but Rome and, by who else but a woman, Fabiola.[1] However, it took many decades before the hospitals in Europe attained anything close to the comprehensive approach and professional care of those in the East.

CONCLUSION

The intended scope of this book is not to elucidate the entire journey from the care provided by monasteries in Europe to the hospitals of the Middle Ages and to those of the modern day. Rather, it is to call out and emphasize the linkage between the Catholic Church and its commitment to offer physical healing, especially to the poor, and to underscore that this connection between the Church and hospitals is theologically and scripturally based, robust and essential, and a societal expectation throughout many centuries.

The question this leaves us with as we continue to examine Catholic healthcare is this: "Has this understanding and commitment been honored and sustained by the current Catholic healthcare system in America?"

CHAPTER 2

The Beginnings of Catholic Healthcare in America

Blessed are the merciful, for they will be shown mercy.
                                                       Jesus, Matthew 5:7

The Catholic healthcare system in America began with the arrival of 12 French Ursuline Sisters in New Orleans, Louisiana, in 1727. Within a few months of their arrival, they were caring for many in need. Before the decade had ended, they had established a hospital. "*In their desire to make themselves useful, they made themselves indispensable.*"[1] This could be said of all the orders of women religious, often called sisters or nuns, who created the foundation of and the model for Catholic healthcare in America.

Unlike the central role the religious orders of women played in establishing Catholic healthcare, the religious orders of men, some of whom had a healthcare focus in Europe, had considerably less involvement in establishing hospitals in America.

Over the next two centuries, the efforts and commitment of nuns in caring for those in need produced the Catholic healthcare system and influenced the evolution of American healthcare. Many books and histories from the various religious orders paint a surprising, often exciting, tale of the work of individual nuns and their religious communities in this effort. One such beautiful and inspiring book, *A Call to Care: The Women Who Built Catholic Healthcare in America*, depicts those contributions in words and pictures and provides a rich resource for much of the following information[1] (permission granted, The Catholic Health Association of the United States).

The stories of nuns' personal sacrifice, including the sacrifice of their own lives, are an inspiration. They clearly were the Good Samaritans of their day in caring for those in need, especially those whom society ignored, marginalized, or persecuted. Like the biblical Good Samaritan, they were often viewed with suspicion in a country that for many decades had harbored mistrust or even dislike of Catholics.

Service being administered to those in need by these women in their unique attire (habits) became the image of the Catholic Church in America. They laid a strong foundation for the American Catholic Church in healthcare and education. Through 800 hospitals and 10,000 schools these women established in cities and towns across the nation, they not only provided healthcare and education to thousands, but made these institutions the bedrock of American Catholicism.[2]

The nuns in the early days of the United States were often "missionaries" from European countries. However, there were soon American offshoots of these orders as well as newly formed American orders. Eventually, there were over 400 hundred orders and chapters of women religious, many of whom were engaged in healthcare (Table 2.1).[1,2]

Healthcare had not been the principal purpose of many religious orders, and for most of the individual nuns, not their training. In fact, these women came to communities to be teachers and start schools. Over the decades, they made an enormous contribution to American education, from grade schools, to colleges, to health professional schools. Education was not to be their sole contribution to the well-being of Americans, however. Soon, they were called upon to serve on battlefields; build and serve in the infirmaries, clinics, and hospitals; and answer the call during epidemics.[1,2,3]

Those who think of nuns as women sheltered behind convent walls, retiring, meek, and withdrawn from the world and its messy issues, should rethink that perception of the nuns who built Catholic healthcare in America.

Many of the founders of the religious orders in the United States had escaped persecution and the convent confinements in Europe to the freedom here. These nuns were courageous, tough, resilient, and entrepreneurial women who did not shy away from any challenge to bring care and caring to those in need.

They walked across deserts to get to a community that needed them, went into mine shafts to provide care, begged in the streets to get needed funds, slept on floors to give beds to patients, wielded hammers to build hospitals, held off mobs with rifles, challenged recalcitrant pastors, bishops, or stagecoach bandits who wanted the money they had collected, and fired surgeons.[1,2,3]

TABLE 2.1. Religious Orders of Nuns Who Started or Administered Hospitals

Adrian Dominican Sisters	Sisters of Humility of Mary
Benedictine Sisters	Sisters of Mary of the Presentation
Benedictine Sisters of Annunciation Monastery	Sisters of Mercy
Benedictine Sisters of Mother of God Monastery	Sisters of Mercy of the Americas
Daughters of Charity	Sisters of Mercy of the Holy Cross
Daughters of Charity of St. Vincent DePaul	Sisters of Misericordia
Dominican Sisters	Sisters of Providence
Dominican Sisters of Peace	Sisters of St. Agnes
Dominican Sisters of St. Catherine of Siena	Sisters of St. Dominic, Congregation of the Most Holy Rosary
Felician Sisters	Sisters of St. Francis
Franciscan Sisters of Allegany	Sisters of St. Francis of Colorado Springs
Franciscan Sisters of Little Falls, Minnesota	Sisters of St. Francis of Our Lady of Lourdes
Franciscan Sisters of Mary	Sisters of St. Francis of Penance and Christian Charity
Franciscan Sisters of Perpetual Adoration	Sisters of St. Francis of Philadelphia
Franciscan Sisters of the Poor	Sisters of St. Francis Seraph of Perpetual Adoration
French Ursuline	Sisters of St. Francis of the Immaculate Heart of Mary
Maryknoll Sisters	Sisters of St. Joseph
Missionary Sisters of the Sacred Heart	Sisters of St. Joseph of Carondelet
Poor Handmaids of Jesus Christ	Sisters of St. Joseph of Nazareth
Presentation Sisters	Sisters of St. Joseph of Orange
Religious Hospitallers of St. Joseph	Sisters of St. Joseph of Peace
Sisters of Bon Secours	Sisters of St. Joseph of the Third Order of St. Francis
Sisters of Charity	Sisters of St. Joseph of Wheeling
Sisters of Charity of Cincinnati	Sisters of St. Joseph of Wichita
Sisters of Charity of Leavenworth	Sisters of St. Mary of the Third Order of St. Francis
Sisters of Charity of Ottawa	Sisters of the Holy Family of Nazareth
Sisters of Charity of St. Elizabeth	Sisters of the Presentation of the Blessed Virgin Mary
Sisters of Charity of the Incarnate Word	Sisters of the Sorrowful Mother
Sisters of Charity of Nazareth	Sylvania Franciscans
Sisters of the Holy Cross	

Derived from Farren S. *A Call to Care: The Women Who Built Catholic Healthcare in America*. St. Louis, Missouri: Catholic Health Association of United States; 1996.
www.commonspirit.org/who-we-are/our-history

They did not turn their faces, their hands, or their hearts from the blood-drenched battlefield, the deformed face of a leper, the stench of a tenement, or the suffering of the dying. They were on the frontlines of healthcare. "*They became the first cadre of independent women professionals.*"[2]

In a seeming contradiction to their membership in a religious community still governed by constraints imposed from Rome and the control of bishops, the nuns had more autonomy and power than other women of their time, and they used it for good. This autonomy was especially true for those living on the frontier.

> "*Because of the remoteness of the centers of authority and because of the paucity of priests, nursing communities tended to develop their own 'western'-style independent ministry, one that was open, expansive, and conscious of doing prayer in action.*"[4]

RESPONDING TO THE CALL FOR HELP

During the Civil War and, to a lesser extent, in the Spanish-American War, nursing was desperately needed, and the nuns answered the call without hesitation. Although Catholics constituted only about 10% of the population of the United States at this time, nuns from 12 orders comprised 20% of the nursing force during the Civil War, numbering over 600.[5] They cared for injured soldiers from both sides on the battlefields, in field tents and in hospitals (Figure 2.1).[1,2,3,4] Serving in the war did not mesh with many of the rules, regulations, and religious practices that nuns usually were expected to follow. A leader of the Sisters of St. Joseph of Philadelphia responded to those concerns with this appraisal:

> "*Go to Holy Communion when you have that favor...Make your meditation in the morning after your prayers and be not troubled if you can say no other prayers of the community, not even if you are deprived of Mass on Sundays...Offer up all the actions of the day, attend to those poor people and I think Our Lord will be satisfied.*"[3]

Some priests and bishops did not always share this view or the nuns' zeal for helping the soldiers at the expense of traditional rituals. They appeared to be more concerned about the maintenance of rules and regulations than mercy — a bit reminiscent of those who passed by the traveler in the parable of the Good Samaritan (see Chapter 1).

For example, the priest who oversaw a group of the Daughters of Charity refused to allow them to serve on hospital transport boats, which desperately needed nurses, because they could not go to Mass or receive

Chapter 2: The Beginnings of Catholic Healthcare in America | 23

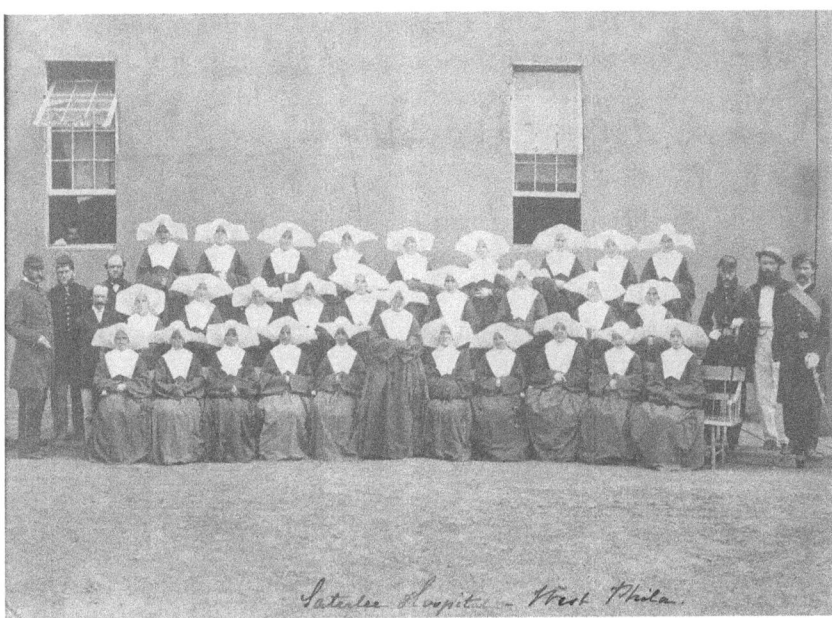

Figure 2.1. Daughters of Charity at the Satterlee Hospital during the Civil War.
Image courtesy of the Archives of the Daughters of Charity Province of St. Louis, St. Louis, MO

communion since there was no priest on board.[3] The Archbishop of New York objected to the Daughters of Charity offering to send up to 100 nurses to serve in the war.[3] This would not be the last time the nuns and Church hierarchy had a differing view of the meaning of serving God.

Many a suffering soldier saw the gift the nuns offered. One Civil War soldier's diary captures what the nuns did:

> *"Amid a sea of blood she performed the most revolting duties for those poor soldiers. She seemed like a ministering angel, and many a young soldier owes his life to her care and charity."*[1]

After visiting one hospital that the nuns staffed, President Lincoln noted:

> *"Of all the forms of charity and benevolence seen in the crowded wards of the hospitals, those of the Catholic Sisters were among the most efficient."*[2]

Some of the nuns who served until the end of the war were taken as prisoners of war and detained for months.[3] In recognition of all the care and caring these nurses provided to soldiers on both sides, a monument was erected in Washington, DC, in 1924 that depicts different orders of nuns. The inscriptions read:

> *(At the top of the relief)*: "They comforted the dying, nursed the wounded, carried hope to the imprisoned, gave in his name a drink of water to the thirsty" *(Beneath the relief)*: "To the memory and in honor of the various orders of sisters who gave their services as nurses on battlefields and in hospitals during the Civil War"[6]

Just as the care provided by early Christians to both Christians and non-Christians contributed to the growth of the Church (see Chapter 1), the selfless, merciful caring the nuns gave to the wounded helped to quell some of the anti-Catholic sentiment of the time. When an old man was checking into Gettysburg's hotel to find his son after that horrific battle, he saw the Daughters of Charity caring for the wounded. He said,

"Good God, can those Sisters be the persons whose religion we always run down? The owner replied, Yes...they are the very persons who are run down by those who know nothing of their charity."[7]

This commitment to serve in times of crisis was not limited to answering the call during conflicts. Just as the early Christians cared for the victims of the plague, the nuns cared for victims of cholera, smallpox, yellow fever, and influenza during the many epidemics that befell American cities.[2,3] They often did what no others could be persuaded to do. During these epidemics, many nuns lost their lives in the service of others.

Their care of cholera victims in 1855 in San Francisco elicited this observation:

> "The Sisters of Mercy, rightly named...did not stop to inquire whether the poor sufferers were Protestants or Catholics, Americans or foreigners, but with the noblest devotion applied themselves to their relief...the idea of dangers never seems to have occurred to these noble women."[2]

The patients for whom they cared during these epidemics were grateful—the sisters' only earthly reward. One resident of Mississippi, where the Sisters of Mercy volunteered to care for yellow fever patients, expressed her gratitude:

"Day and night they were by our bedsides, trying to comfort us, to gratify our wishes .... A mother could not have done more or been more self-sacrificing than were these good Sisters."[3]

During a smallpox epidemic in Texas in 1891, they even lived in the same "pest house" with the victims.[1] Their care of smallpox victims in New York City elicited the following comment from a city leader:

"No one can witness the faithfulness and self-sacrifice with which these pious women discharge their duties, regardless of their own comfort, and intent only on the welfare of those entrusted to their care...."[1]

Not every city leader was as grateful for their commitment. After they had worked tirelessly in San Francisco during the 1855 cholera epidemic, the city's board of supervisors refused to pay them what was owed.[2] But the city underestimated Mother Russell, the Sister of Mercy leading the community in San Francisco — not the first or the last group to be outmaneuvered by a nun. She canceled the contract to run the hospital, bought it, and reopened it as St. Mary's, which became one of the foundations of what is now CommonSpirit, one of the largest Catholic healthcare systems in America.[2]

Moreover, despite the lauds and expressions of gratitude the nuns received, they had to face anti-Catholic sentiment even as they nursed on battlefields and in the cities.[4] They were the target of the Klu Klux Klan and the Know Nothings.[2] In fact, a mob burned down a school in Massachusetts in 1834, killing one sister.[2]

In the 1800s and 1900s, nuns from the religious orders outnumbered the priests. With their habits flying behind them, they fanned out across the country answering the calls of bishops, miners, lumberjacks, farmers, immigrants, and cities to start hospitals in their communities.

By the mid-1920s, the nuns were operating 500 hospitals; by 1928, there were more than 600 Catholic hospitals in America.[3,4] Often, these hospitals were the first hospitals in the territory or the state. They were in major cities from New York City to San Francisco and small towns from Altoona, Pennsylvania, to Aberdeen, South Dakota.[1,2,3]

While the nuns opened many hospitals across the United States to serve immigrants who were often not welcomed in the hospitals at the time, these hospitals largely served European immigrants. How non-European immigrants and Native Americans were served in the emerging Catholic hospitals of the late 1800s and early 1900s is less clear. Were their doors open to all those who came to them?

CATHOLIC HOSPITALS AND BLACK AMERICANS

There was at least one group of Americans to whom the door to the hospitals appeared only slightly ajar—black Americans. How wide open that door was and where the women religious stood on race issues is a mixed picture. While there are noteworthy exceptions, it seems that in large part, Catholic hospitals reflected American society's view of race and (in)equality at any given time. Sadly, a number of women religious communities had owned slaves or profited from the labor of slaves.[8,9] However, the women religious from the Sisters of Charity Federation acknowledge this history and the need for forgiveness and change:

> "Yet, while the institution of slavery and the exploitation of enslaved people was deeply engrained in society and the economy of the 19th century, this shameful historical reality does not diminish our profound regret and dismay today. We, who follow in the footsteps of the original Sisters of Charity of St. Joseph and the Daughters of Charity of St. Vincent de Paul in the United States apologize and ask for forgiveness....We pledge to move further into the work of racial equity; to remember and learn from our past; and confront systemic racism through our words and actions."[10]

By the early 1900s, only about 2.0% of the 12 million black Americans were Catholics and there were only a few black priests and only two orders of black nuns.[2,3,4] A black journalist and activist, Daniel Rudd, sought to change that and formed a group called the Black Catholic Congress with the belief that the Catholic Church, in fact, could be a pivotal ally in the fight for justice and equality.[11]

The group held a series of meetings and solicited input from every American bishop regarding the occurrence of discrimination in their dioceses. In response to that survey, a statement was issued at the 1894 meeting opposing racial discrimination within Catholic institutions, primarily in schools, but also in Catholic hospitals.[4] This plea to end discrimination was largely unheeded, at least in regard to hospitals.

Kauffman noted that in 1925, Floyd Keeler, in his book *Catholic Medical Missions*, stated, "*everywhere the Catholic hospitals exist provision is made for the admission of colored patients and the contact with the Catholic sister nurse, priest or doctor is all that could be given under the circumstance.*"[4] In fact, those circumstances may have been quite constrained.

According to Kauffman, a Jesuit priest, John T. Gillard, detailed a 1928 survey, saying, "*While no information is available as to how many of the 612 Catholic hospitals provide bed space for Negroes, it is definitely known that many of them refuse their ministration to Negroes.*"[4]

On the other side of the coin, some of the orders of nuns opened hospitals in a number of cities, including in the South, specifically to serve the black communities. By the mid-1940s, there were nine such hospitals.[3,4] In 1941, the Sisters of Mercy opened Saint Martin de Porres Hospital in Mobile, Alabama, for black patients, including a one-room maternity ward.[12] It operated until 1971, when a separate facility was no longer needed.[12] The largest such black patient-serving hospital was St. Mary's Infirmary in St. Louis, which in 1945 had 150 beds.[4] It was also the first hospital open to black physicians.[4]

Concurrent with these efforts to establish separate but segregated facilities were initial efforts to integrate hospitals. In 1946, the Sisters of St. Joseph of the Third Order of St. Francis opened St. Joseph Hospital in Meridian, Mississippi, stating they would accept black and white patients. This was not well-received by the community.

The Sisters stated that ambulances would bypass their hospital, only bringing them *"patients who couldn't pay."*[1] The passage of time and even the Civil Rights legislation did not seem to change the views of the Meridian community, for when the nuns there fed the students who came to Mississippi to rebuild a burnt black church, they were boycotted, and the following message was distributed in the community:

> *"Attention white citizens of Meridian and Lauderdale County. Listed below are a few people and businesses who are traitors and parasites, who would sell their souls for thirty pieces of silver—integration."*[1]

The hospital was considered one such parasite and it almost failed as a result of this, but the Sisters hung on.

In the late 1940s, under the direction of the Archbishop of Washington, DC, Georgetown Hospital offered integrated floors and open admissions, but the segregated semiprivate and four-bed rooms remained.[4] In 1953, the bishop of Kansas City opened an integrated hospital — integrated for patients and physicians. At his Labor Day Mass, he stated:

> *"This is my message to Kansas City....no longer to deny intelligent Negro doctors the opportunity of employment of their skilled profession....Kansas City must provide without delay accredited and properly equipped hospital facilities in which competent Negro physicians may work side by side with white members of their profession in promoting the health of this community."*[4]

There were a few other notable Catholic hospitals that integrated staff. In 1951, when Sister Helen Clare, who was running St. Francis Hospital in Wheeling, West Virginia, refused to fire three black nurses, 20 white nurses, and some physicians quit in protest for having to work with black nurses.[1] Sister Helen Clare airlifted other Sisters of St. Joseph into the hospital to provide staff. The census went down, but the hospital survived. Sister Helen Clare stayed true to her belief:

> *"As a Catholic institution it will continue to uphold Christian principles of charity and justice as well as the spirit of the United States Constitution."*[1]

Despite the examples in Kansas and West Virginia, the Catholic hospitals in the South, and even some in the North, were segregated for both staff and patients, as were the non-Catholic hospitals. Whether it was the nuns' decision or the decision of others to maintain segregated hospitals is not known. However, after the passage of the Civil Rights legislation of 1964 and the establishment of Medicare and Medicaid in 1965, such segregation was illegal if those government payments were made to the hospitals.

In this time of civil rights awakening in America, the nuns were highly engaged. Some historians would say *"it was the Catholic sisters who finally brought home to the average Catholic the message of racial tolerance."*[2]

They led marches in Chicago and New York. They were marching in Selma, and they cared for the injured there.[2]

In 2018, the United States Conference of Catholic Bishops released an important pastoral letter on racism: *Open Wide Our Hearts*.[13] It addresses racism among all groups, not just African Americans. It concludes with several notable statements:

> *"Therefore, we, the Catholic bishops of the United States, acknowledge the many times when the Church has failed to live as Christ taught — to love our brothers and sisters. Acts of racism have been committed by leaders and members of the Catholic Church — by bishops, clergy, religious, and laity — and her institutions. We express deep sorrow and regret for them. We also acknowledge those instances when we have not done enough or stood by silently when grave acts of injustice were committed. We ask for forgiveness from all who have been harmed by these sins committed in the past or in the present.... Consequently, we all need to take responsibility for correcting the injustices of racism and healing the harms it has caused."*[13]

ENABLING THE CARE

The nuns relied heavily on donations to open and operate every hospital. They could keep operating costs considerably lower than could other hospitals because the nuns did not receive salaries and their existence was a frugal one, as most religious orders took vows of poverty. The donations were both monetary and in kind — some rather unusual: a cow arriving by steamship in Vancouver with a tag "For Mother Joseph" and a pork chop thrown at the begging nuns to get rid of them. The pork chop was considered a donation, picked up, washed off, and eaten for dinner.[1,14]

The nuns often "made the rounds," collecting donations door to door, business to business, and from mining camps to lumber camps. They were quite innovative, even obtaining tax deductions from counties and cities for their services.[1] One very clever investment entailed employing laid-off railroad workers to build and run a sawmill to supply railroad ties to the railroads and using the income to build and run a hospital to care for the railroad workers.[1] The nuns understood win-win-win before it was a concept!

The nuns even started the first prepaid health insurance plans.[1,15] A lumberjack in the Wisconsin woods could pay five dollars for a "lumberjack ticket" which would entitle him to treatment in the hospital in Tomahawk for one year.[1,14,15] If only insurance were that cheap and easy to obtain today!

Operating hospitals not only requires money, but also trained personnel. Again, the women religious responded, uniting their historical roles as educators and caregivers by starting nursing schools. This helped to develop nursing as a profession, created a pipeline for the women who are the backbone of healthcare delivery, and established a path for upward mobility for women, and especially immigrant women.[16]

At the end of the 1800s, there were about 20 Catholic nursing schools. By 1915, there were 220 Catholic nursing schools training nuns and lay women.[3] Today, 155 Catholic nursing schools in the United States continue to train the nurses that staff the hospitals, the clinics, and all the venues where they serve.[17]

While the nuns fervently embraced Catholicism, they had a deep understanding of America's pluralistic society and the boundaries that it created. This is reflected in Mother Clark's instruction manual for nurses written in 1841:

> *"...a sister should greet new patients first with physical comforts and then say, 'of what religion are you?.... If he says, 'I am a*

Protestant' — *she should say nothing more but give him all the temporal assistance he needs.*"[4]

The Metropolitan Catholic Almanac's description of the care provided by the Sisters of Charity at St. John's Infirmary in Milwaukee in 1850 stated:

"Any patient may call for any clergyman he may prefer...but no minister...will be permitted to interfere religiously with, such patients as do not ask for the exercise of his office. The rights of conscience must be held paramount to all others."[4]

CATHOLIC HOSPITALS AND COMMUNITY PHYSICIANS

While the nuns opened and managed the hospitals and provided much of the caring, they were not the physicians. The physicians came from the community and were paid or chose to practice at the hospitals.[1,3,4] Although one would expect a range of impressions and interactions between the women religious and the mostly male physicians, it appears to have largely been one of mutual respect — even protection!

Sister Stanislaus at Charity Hospital in New Orleans wrote to another sister in 1913:

"...we are sort of a mystery to these new doctors. They cannot understand our lives. The untiring devotedness and sincere interest by our sisters in their various duties puzzles them." She went on to note: *"Two doctors ...wonder(ed) (that Sister) must get a goodly salary for running that place."*[1]

One of the Sisters of Providence from St. Vincent Hospital in Portland understood and embraced the critical role of the physicians in building the hospitals, noting in the yearly report in 1875 that:

"It was his [Dr. Kinney's] skill that really made the reputation of the hospital." [14]

There is an amazing story of a nun who bargained with Billy the Kid to save four physicians' scalps.[2] A Sister of Mercy, Sister Blandina, working in the rough and tumble town of Trinidad, Colorado, witnessed a gunfight involving one of Billy the Kid's gang members.[2] Having been shot in the leg, Schneider was thrown into an abandoned hut to die, but Sister Blandina came to nurse him, unintimidated by his telling her stories of his acts of violence.[2]

Chapter 2: The Beginnings of Catholic Healthcare in America | **31**

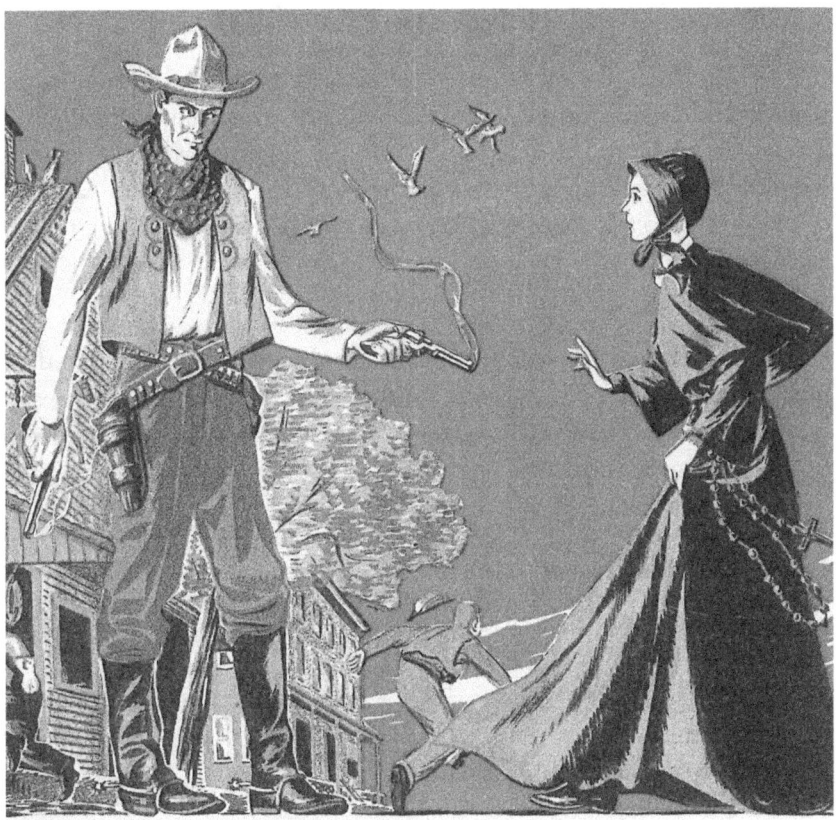

Figure 2.2. Illustration of the Encounter of Sister Blandina with Billy the Kid: Illustration of Sister Blandina, a Sister of Charity, encountering Billy the Kid while working in Trinidad, Colorado.
Image courtesy of the Sisters of Charity of Cincinnati Archives Department. Sister Blandina Seagle Special Collection: Article Relevant, Committed, Liberated Sisters Always with Us by S. Marie Emmanuel, SC, printed in Immaculata (1976).

On one of her visits, Billy the Kid was there and threatened to scalp the four doctors who had refused to treat Schneider. We are not privy to the exact exchange but apparently in return for the care she had given to his gang member, he said, "*It would be a pleasure to be able to do you any favor.*"[2] "The Kid" met his match because she asked the doctors to be spared, which "the Kid" did[2] — the power of one nun! (Figure 2.2)

The mutual respect, trust, and commitment to work together across disciplines and faiths was demonstrated dramatically by Mother Alfred and Dr. W.W Mayo. She provided the nurses and the hospital, and he provided physician expertise without any legal contract — such was the birth of the Mayo Clinic.[2]

NUNS IN A MAN'S WORLD

Just as with the nuns who headed to the frontier to start hospitals, the women leading religious orders and healthcare institutions were allowed a degree of autonomy and authority that was not afforded the women in the overall society. This period when the nuns were building the network of Catholic hospitals was not a time when men in the Church or in society took direction from women leaders. (One can legitimately ask, "Is now such a time?")

The nuns were part of society and a Catholic hierarchy dominated by men. But they were on a mission, and they exerted authority when necessary. Anyone who has fired a surgeon for failure to follow the rules will find this example impressive:

Mother Valencia ran St. Francis Hospital in Hartford, Connecticut. When a respected surgeon refused to come into the hospital in the middle of the night to operate on a poor old woman, she called him to her office and fired him, telling him, "*We have no stars here.*"[1]

She and the others like her who did not shrink from defending what was right and needed must have believed Mother Clare Cusack: "*The future of the world will be what women make it.*"[1]

Some bishops supported the sisters' efforts. Others were not only unhelpful, they were obstructive. Following their vows of obedience, the sisters at times bowed to the bishops' directives. But they also confronted the bishops and used their power and autonomy, sometimes moving to another city with a more supportive bishop to provide care for the new dioceses.[1,2]

There were bishops such as Bishop John Carroll of Maryland, the first bishop in America, who was a great support for Mother Elizabeth Seton and shared her ideas about the role and work of nuns in this new country.[18] Bishop Michael O'Connor clearly saw what the nuns could offer to this new country and even traveled to Ireland to bring sisters to help in the emerging frontier town of Pittsburgh.[2] He became a lifelong friend of Mother Frances Warde, who established the Sisters of Mercy, the largest American order.[2]

But some bishops (some would say the majority) sought to constrain the nuns or even demand that they abide by the old restrictions, including living in convents, requiring permission for almost any activity, and following the bishops' orders. The nuns, especially those in the western United

States, were quite independent, even riding horseback into the wilderness. However, over time, this freedom was rescinded.

When the Catholic Hospital Association (now the Catholic Health Association) was formed, in large part by the efforts of the Sisters of St. Joseph of Carondelet, the bishops prohibited nuns from serving as officers, a situation which lasted from 1915 to the 1960s.[1,19] These re-emerged constraints may have contributed to the dwindling number of nuns in America (see Chapter 7). One sister in recent times noted, *"I am responsible for a $3 million budget, but I can't drive to a meeting at night without special permission."*[3]

Pittsburgh's Bishop Domenec, a quite different bishop than Bishop O'Connor, ordered a re-organization of the sisters of Mercy, telling them if they resisted, *"...then the community will suffer...on account of your resistance to lawful authority."*[2] He lost his position; the pope was on the side of the nuns this time, but that was not always the case. There were bishops like Bishop James Oliver Van de Velde who believed sisters had no right to own property — property they had worked hard to obtain — and demanded the deeds to their lakeside Chicago property.[2] He did not get those deeds.

One famous diocesan move was made by Mother Alfred, who was removed from her leadership role by another bishop of Chicago. Not to be put down, she took 23 of her nuns and moved to Rochester, Minnesota. There, she led St. Mary's Hospital and later partnered with Dr. W.W. Mayo.[2] It seems like Mother Alfred and Rochester won that tussle. The nuns may have been victorious not only on earth, but also, perhaps, in heaven, as six American nuns have been canonized as saints.

CONCLUSION

During the period when the nuns were building Catholic healthcare in America as well as now, the bishops who made decisions and issued directives often lived in relative comfort and rarely, if ever, were on battlefields, in tenements, mining camps, leper colonies, or hospitals tending the sick. The nuns who saw and cared for the sick were then and now the voices of those in need. When that required them to disagree with the bishops, they did and continue to do so.

In 2010, the bishops opposed the Affordable Care Act and the nuns supported it.[19,20] The nuns' support reflected their role in providing care: *"As the heads of major Catholic women's religious order in the United States, we represent 59,000 Catholic Sisters in the United States who respond to needs of people in many ways... We have witnessed firsthand the impact of our national health care crises, particularly its impact on women, children, and people who are poor."*[20]

The bishops issued a letter opposing gender-affirming care while the nuns issued a very different letter of support for these patients (see Chapter 5). The bishops and many leaders of Catholic healthcare today have never cared for the sick and suffering directly. This lived experience is missing and must have an influence on their perspectives, thinking, and leadership.

CHAPTER 3

Exemplary Mothers

I feel an irresistible force drawing me to follow this call.
Mother Marianne Cope

Leaders of the women religious orders, typically referred to as "Mother" or "Mother Superior," often were the ones who opened or managed hospitals in the early days of American healthcare — they were the CEOs. They are an inspiration — especially for women leaders and those who still see healthcare as a calling and not a business.

Although one could tell many hundreds of inspiring stories about these women leaders, I chose five exemplary Mothers who were inspiring and remarkably different from each other. Nuns were not cookie-cutter personas. Their varying skills and approaches paint the rich picture of the foundations of Catholic healthcare.

Yet, as different as they were, they all embodied zeal, resilience, tenacity, faith, hope, sacrificial caring, and compassion. They stand as role models and mirrors of self-reflection for current leaders of Catholic healthcare and, in fact, for all healthcare leaders.

MOTHER MARIANNE COPE

Mother Marianne Cope's story told here is taken from *A Song of Pilgrimage and Exile,* unless otherwise indicated.[1] She was born Barbara Koop to a Catholic family in Germany in 1838. In 1840, her parents emigrated to Utica, New York, where she grew up in a large family of very modest means. In 1862, she entered religious life into the Third Order of St. Francis at their convent in Syracuse, New York (Figure 3.1). She rose through the leadership of the Order and in 1870 found herself as the leader of the newly opened St. Joseph's Hospital in Syracuse. In 1877, she was elected the leader of her religious community.

While these roles were challenging, they did not compare to the stark realities that awaited her. A June 1883 letter from a missionary priest begged

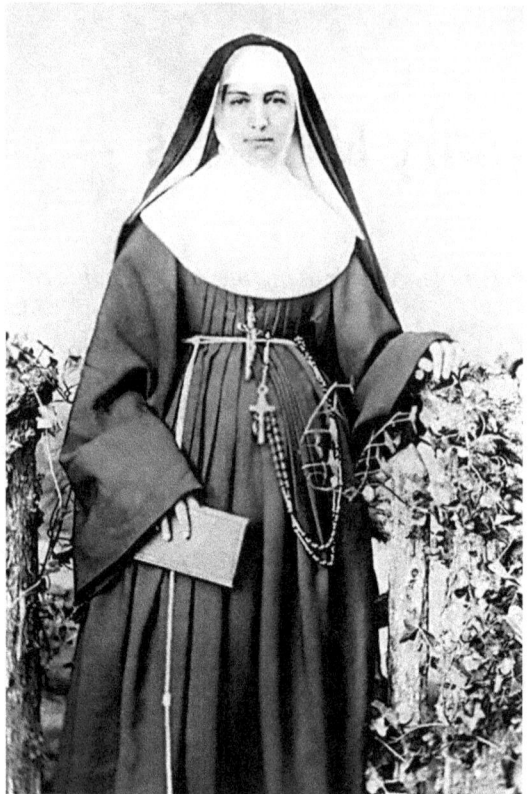

Figure 3.1. Mother Marianne Cope, a nun of Sisters of the Third Order of Saint Francis, who worked, lived, and died for the lepers in Hawaii.
Image Wikipedia: Public Domain

her to bring sisters to Hawaii to care for the sick. This letter changed her life. Her response to the letter was,

"Shall I regard your kind invitation to join you in your missionary labors, as coming from God....I feel an irresistible force drawing me to follow this call...."[1]

At the time, 50 orders of religious were asked to come to Hawaii for this work and only Mother Marianne and her community responded.[2]

In November, she came face to face with the reality of this call when she entered the Branch Hospital in Kakaako, Hawaii, which housed the lepers:

"...permeating everything — air, clothes, straw pallets, greasy blankets, even the wood of the walls and the dirt on the floors — hung the stink of

lepers: *the revolting stench rising from the sores, unwashed and uncovered, the miasma of dead and rotting flesh.... Mother Marianne saw, smelled, heard, felt all those horrors....*"[1]

But unlike what almost all of us would do, she and the other sisters who came with her did not turn away, never to return. Perhaps she had cemented in her mind a picture of Jesus touching and healing the lepers, or she recalled St. Francis, who got down from his horse and embraced and kissed the leper as a brother despite his initial revulsion.

The six nuns began scrubbing away years of dirt on everything from the pots in the kitchen to the walls of the cottages. Then they cleaned the lepers' wounds. The commitment this required is underscored by the fact that some sisters from her order who came later did not stay.

The situation Mother Marianne found at the Branch Hospital clearly showed that the current leadership was inadequate. When she asked for clarification of her authority, she was told that the nun's work was "women's work," and women's work did not include leadership — or so some thought. Months later, she called a meeting with the three men who were obstructing her mission to care for the lepers: the steward of the hospital, a political leader, and the bishop. "*Behind the serene countenance...hid a will of tempered steel....*"[1] She informed them she and her sisters would not stay if her conditions were not met. The outcome is easily deduced.

She had promised her sisters that none would contract leprosy and neither she nor they did.[2]

Mother Marianne cared for the lepers for 35 years, from 1883 to her death in 1918, first at Branch Hospital and then in the leper colony at Molokai.[1] In recognition of this astounding commitment, she has been called the "*beloved mother of the outcasts.*"[2]

She was canonized a saint of the Catholic Church in 2012 by Pope Benedict XVI. At the canonization, the pope said, "*At a time when little could be done for those suffering from this terrible disease, Marianne Cope showed the highest love, courage, and enthusiasm. She is a shining and energetic example of the best of the tradition of Catholic nursing sisters and of the spirit of her beloved Saint Francis.*"[2]

MOTHER FRANCIS CABRINI

As a daughter in an Italian immigrant family, I must tell the story of Mother Francis Cabrini (Figure 3.2). The details of her journey are

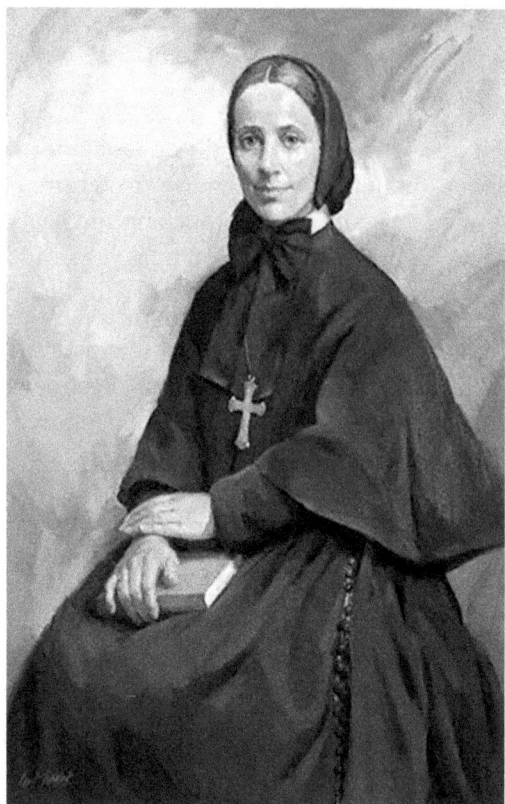

Figure 3.2. Mother Francis Cabrini founded the Missionary Sisters of the Sacred Heart, who established schools and hospitals throughout the Americas.
Image courtesy of the Mother Cabrini Shrine, Golden Colorado

presented in the *Immigrant Saint*; the following information is taken from that source unless otherwise noted.[3]

Born Francesca Maria Cabrina in rural Italy in 1850, she was so frail that she was rejected by the Daughters of the Sacred Heart as not strong enough to do the work of a nun. She was not to be deterred. In 1880, she recruited seven orphans and began her own religious order, the Missionary Sisters of the Sacred Heart. This foreshadowed her undeterred zeal for her work.

At the pope's personal direction, she was led not to China as she had planned, but to America. She left her mark in the United States and Central and South America, and founded hospitals in New York City, Chicago, and Seattle.

It was during the renovations of Columbus Hospital in Chicago that Mother Cabrini proved herself a force to be reckoned with. The job was in tatters due to contractors' mismanagement: *"Greedy heartless contractors.... The devil of bad faith is in them! This moment I could devour them alive!"*[3]

She figuratively did exactly that, summoning them and demanding they remove their workers and equipment from the site. The response she heard was, *"Lady, just who are you?"* To which she responded in Italian, *"Madre Cabrini, Superiora Generale delle Missionarie del S. Cuore"* — that said it all, even if it was in Italian.[3]

As remarkable as this was, what happened next was even more amazing. She went into the Italian community for whom the hospital was to be a haven and found brick layers, carpenters, and others who volunteered to finish the job under her supervision — no doubt better than it would have been with the original contractors. She opened the hospital in February 1905.[3]

Her commitment to those in need was exemplified not only in the work but in her words of guidance:

> *"Observe unflinchingly the realities of that which causes want, pain, misunderstanding and tragedy. Let us put courageous and probing hands to these injustices and social wounds inflicted on our dear good people."*[3]

Her words of warning about what could deter healthcare from this path of service should be inscribed above the entrance of every Catholic healthcare facility:

> *"We must beware of two temptations, that of failure and that of success; and often prosperity will be more dangerous than adversity."*[3]

Catholic healthcare in America was built by the women religious who vowed poverty and never bowed to the temptation of prosperity. Yet, this temptation is an issue for Catholic healthcare in America today (see Chapter 8).

This woman, who was deemed too frail to join a convent, traveled throughout the United States, crossed the Atlantic 27 times, traveled to Central and South America, and established 67 institutions: orphanages, schools, and hospitals.

As her establishment of orphanages and schools reflects, she especially cared for children.[4] When in December 1917 she learned that the 500 children at her school in Chicago would not have Christmas candy because of the war, she had the sisters scour for candy.[5] Despite being weak, one of her last acts was helping to pack the candy for the children.[5] She died two days later.[5]

Mother Cabrini was canonized a saint of the Catholic Church July 7, 1946, by Pope Pius XII—the first American citizen to receive this honor.[6] He noted, "*We see her, this heroine of modern times, …rising like a star from a humble town in Lombardy, …spreading the warmth of her rays everywhere.*"[6]

Pope Francis, who cares deeply for the plight of immigrants, has said of her, "*Frances understood that modernity would be marked by these immense migrations and uprooted human beings, in a crisis of identity, often desperate and lacking resources to face the society in which they would have to enter.*"[6]

MOTHER JOSEPH

As frail as Mother Cabrini may have been, Mother Joseph was just the opposite (Figure 3.3). Her story is told in *Cornerstone* and many details that follow are from that source, unless otherwise noted.[7]

She was born Esther Pariseau in the Province of Quebec in 1823. Despite being a girl and the third of 12 children in the 1800s, her mother sent her to a boarding school — undoubtedly not a common choice at that time.[8] Not only was her mother apparently ahead of her time in seeing talents in young women, so was her father, a respected carpenter who built coaches.[8] He welcomed his daughter into his shop and taught her construction skills.[8] This combination of education and hands-on skills served Mother Joseph well throughout her life.

In 1843, she joined the Sisters of Charity of Providence (now Sisters of Providence) in Montreal. Her father told the Mother Superior,

"*I bring you my daughter Esther, who wishes to dedicate herself to the religious life.… She can read and write and figure accurately. She can cook and sew and spin and do all manner of housework well. She has learned carpentry from me and can handle tools as well as I can. Moreover, she can plan and supervise the work of others, and I assure you, Madame, she will some day make a very good superior.*"[8]

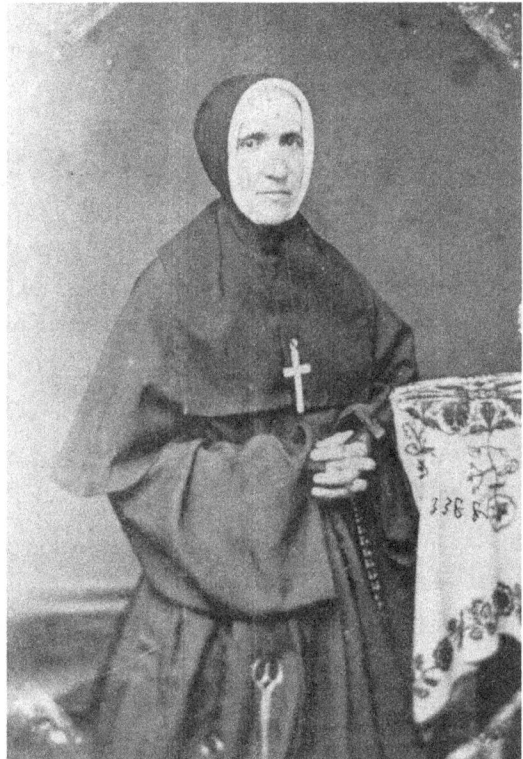

Figure 3.3. Mother Joseph of the Sacred Heart, a Sister of Providence, who established hospitals throughout the Northwest.
Image courtesy of the Providence Archives Seattle, Washington

This was a father who knew his daughter.

In 1856, Mother Joseph and four companions made the difficult journey from Montreal to the Washington Territory. So began her transformative influence on the Pacific Northwest. It is worth noting that she was clearly ahead of her time in seeing the link between education and health, saying, "*Schools are needed first of all.*"[8] She also said, "*Americans do not count the cost where education is concerned.*"[8] If only this were still true.

She built the first hospitals in Washington and Oregon — actually "built."[7] She was an architect and a builder. The images of Mother Joseph are of her striding across the building site with a hammer dangling from her belt, bouncing on a high crossbeam in her habit, or crawling from under a foundation. In 1953, the American Institute of Architects declared Mother Joseph "The First Architect of the Northwest."[9]

Although she demanded quality buildings, her true work was not about buildings. She established 11 hospitals in Washington, Oregon, Idaho, and Montana that became the foundation for the Providence system, which is the fourth largest healthcare system in the United States[10] (see Chapter 7).

As with all the early Catholic hospitals, money was short. Mother Joseph was famous for her "begging tours" in which she would strike out across this wild territory visiting mining and lumber camps to collect donations — always successful financially, but not without incident. Returning from one long trip, she noted they had encountered a pack of hungry wolves and an angry grizzly bear and had a tent fire.[9]

A fellow nun summed up Mother Joseph's many gifts: *"She had the characteristics of genius: incessant work, immense sacrifices, great undertakings, and she never counted the cost to self."*[9]

Mother Joseph died in 1902. Her last words to her sisters were, *"My dear sisters allow me to recommend to you the care of the poor…. Take good care of them…whatever concerns the poor is always our affair."*[8]

Although Mother Joseph was not canonized a saint, she is one of 11 women representing the states and, of course, and the only nun in Congress' Statuary Hall, representing one of Washington state's two members.[8]

MOTHER ODILIA BERGER

Mother Mary Odilia Berger, a German nun, founded the order of the Franciscan Sisters of Mary (SSM) (Figure 3.4), but only at the end of a long and perilous journey that traversed Germany, France, and ended in the United States. Her journey almost ended before it had begun with an unexpected event for a nun.

The first half century of that journey is told in *A Woman for All Times*.[11] Her work in the United States became the foundation of SSM Health which is among the largest American healthcare systems.[10] That part of the story is well presented in the video on the SSM Health website.[12]

She was born Anna Katharina Berger (called Katharina) in Bavaria in 1823.[11] Many of the details that follow are from *A Woman for All Times* unless otherwise noted. At age 30 she became an unwed mother.[5,11] As happened often in those times, the baby was raised by the grandmother, who she thought was her mother; presumably, she believed her mother was her sister.

Chapter 3: Exemplary Mothers | 43

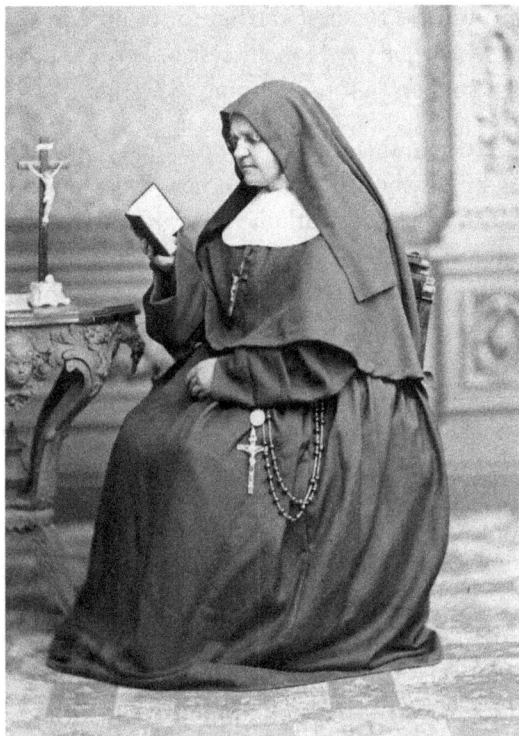

Figure 3.4. Mother Odilia Berger, a Franciscan Sister of Mary, whose work laid the foundation for SSM Health.
Image courtesy of the Franciscan Sisters of Mary Archives

At age 34 having chosen not to marry, Katharina felt called to become a nun. Fortunately for her and American healthcare, a bishop did not see her past and her age as impediments to religious life. Moreover, he agreed that should her daughter require care outside her family, that could be arranged.

In 1858, she joined the Poor Franciscans of Pirmasen. As a nun, she traveled about the countryside and cities, raising funds for the order. Her daughter died in 1864. In 1865, Katharina and another nun were sent to Paris to collect funds and serve the large German community there. Here, her life took another twist.

When she saw young immigrant girls arriving at the train station being pulled unknowingly into a life of prostitution, she wanted to offer them a safe place to start their life in Paris. This may seem a straight-forward path for a nun, but it was not. To start this work, she had to leave the Poor Franciscans. Her hope of starting a new order in Paris was dashed by the onset of the Franco-Prussian war, but the effort earned her the title of Mother Odilia, which she kept for the rest of her life. Escaping Paris, she cared for injured soldiers before returning to Germany.

Once back in Germany, she and her companions began caring for victims of smallpox. Again, she hoped to form a new order, but once more it was not to be. This time, the anti-Catholic government of Bismarck began to threaten her and her companions. Reaching out to a friend whom she had nursed to health and who was now in St. Louis, she obtained a welcome from the bishop to go there. She led a group of five nuns from Germany to St. Louis in 1872 — yet another chapter in her life and one for which she is most remembered. In 1874, she finally formed her order, the Sisters of St. Mary.[11]

Many of the details of her life in St. Louis are from the SSM Health website video.[12] Almost as soon as they set foot in St. Louis, the nuns were caring for the victims of a smallpox epidemic. Because this interaction exposed them to smallpox, they could not travel via public transport, so they walked from house to house. In 1878, the yellow fever epidemic hit the area and the sisters were again called to serve, not only in St. Louis, but also in Tennessee and Mississippi. Many of the young sisters who volunteered for this work died from yellow fever.

Mother Odilia is an example of "servant leadership." She was out in the streets of St. Louis begging. Although she relied heavily on one-on-one generosity, as many of the women religious leaders did, she also had a savvy understanding of capital financing.

Since their arrival, the sisters had been caring for the sick in their homes, which was difficult. Moreover, the 15 hospitals in St. Louis apparently did not open wide their doors to the poor and immigrants. The sisters realized they needed a hospital to shelter and properly nurse as many patients as possible.

Mother Odilia took note of a large vacant house that would serve their needs and welcome those who were unwelcomed by others. The price tag was $16,000 (SSM archivist, personal communication). She knew she would not get this sum of money begging for pennies. Like Willie Sutton who famously said he robbed banks because that was where the money was, she went to the bank, albeit not to rob it. However, the banker may have thought there were some similarities. Not surprisingly, the banker, who was not in the business of charity, said that the bank would want to be paid back and he doubted that the sisters could find that kind of money. He asked, "*Is there someone who will help you assume the responsibility?*"[12] Mother Odilia replied, also not surprisingly, "*St. Joseph will be our security. He has never let us down....*"[12] The banker replied, quite surprisingly, "*With such good backing..., I would be foolish to refuse you.*"[12]

St. Mary's Infirmary opened in 1877. Many patients whom the hospital would subsequently serve had no means to pay and were registered as ODL — Our Dear Lord. If only ODL could be the guarantor for many of the poor in Catholic hospitals today. Additional hospitals were opened in four states.

Mother Odilia died in 1880. Her biographer said of her, "*She was a mixture of humility and weakness, courage, hard-headedness, indestructibility and above all love — a woman for all times.*"[11] She was not canonized and did not have a statue in the halls of Congress, but she was rewarded by the legacy of the network of hospitals that became SSM.

MOTHER ELIZABETH SETON

Last is the improbable journey of Elizabeth Ann Seton, whose history is well known to me from having attended Seton Hill College (now Seton Hill University). Her story is told in the *American Saint* and deserves recounting because of its twists and turns and the work of the religious order she founded. Many of the details that follow are from that source unless otherwise noted.[13] She was rich and poor, Episcopal and Catholic, married and a nun, a mother, and a Mother Superior!

Elizabeth was born Elizabeth Ann Bayley in New York in 1774, about the same time that the United States was born. Her father was a physician and although her family was prosperous, life at that time in America and in her own family was somewhat chaotic, starting with the death of her mother when she was about two years old. At age 16, she met Will Seton and married him at age 20 (Figure 3.5). Will ran a shipping business that had been successful under his father, but it failed, as did his health, from the ravages of tuberculosis which plagued the family and many others in America at that time.

In 1803, Elizabeth and Will and one of their five children departed for Italy, hoping Will's health would improve there. That was not to be; he died in Italy.

Her underlying religious faith and her exposure to Catholicism in Italy led Elizabeth to convert to Catholicism from the Episcopal Church in 1805.

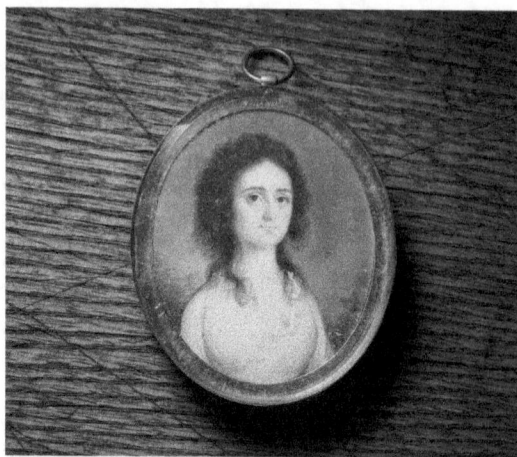

Figure 3.5. A miniature of Elizabeth Seton painted on ivory around the time of her wedding.
Image courtesy of the Seton Shrine at Emmitsburg, Maryland

At that time, she was back in America, a widow responsible for five children. But she had the good fortune of an Italian benefactor as well as a friend in the Bishop of Baltimore who led her to Baltimore and ultimately to a donated, dilapidated farm in Emmitsburg, Maryland. There, with a small group of other women, including some family members and even her daughters, she launched what would be her legacy and her contribution to American Catholicism.

In 1809, she formed the first American women's religious community, the Sisters of Charity of St. Joseph, stating she had *"the joy of my soul at the prospect of being able to assist the poor, visit the sick, comfort the sorrowful, clothe little innocents, and teach them to love God!"*[14] (Figure 3.6).

In 1810, this new sisterhood opened St. Joseph's Academy, a free school for girls, launching their long commitment to the education of children, especially girls. In 1821, Elizabeth Seton died from the same disease that took her husband and two of their children, but the Sisters of Charity continued to grow and serve.

In July 1863, the battle of Gettysburg raged almost on their doorstep and the nuns at Emmitsburg responded to help care for the 45,000 casualties of the battle, staffing St. Francis Xavier Church in Gettysburg, which became a hospital. A beautiful stained-glass window was erected in recognition of their many hours of tireless work with the wounded. The plaque reads:

"During the Battle in Gettysburg this house of God became a hospital for the wounded soldiers. Within its hallowed walls brave men of the North and South foes on the field of battle through weeks of pain were nursed with tender and equal care by the Sisters of Charity of Emmitsburg."[15]

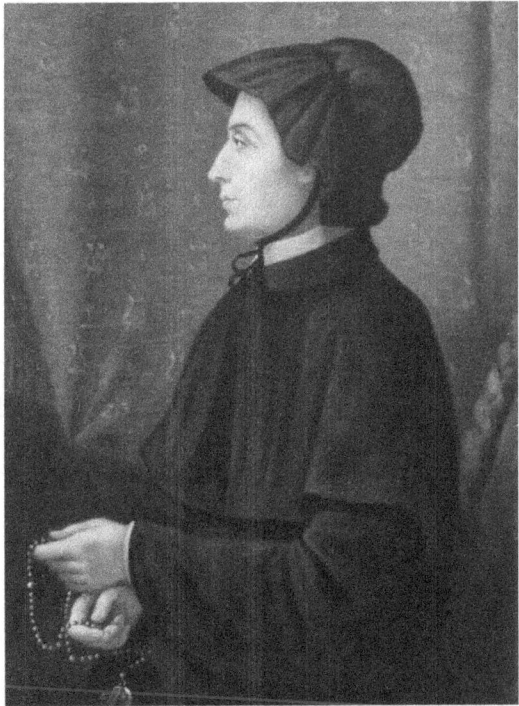

Figure 3.6. Mother Elizabeth Seton, who formed the first American women's religious community, the Sisters of Charity of St. Joseph.
Image courtesy of Daughters of Charity Province of St. Louis, St. Louis MO.

This was not their first or last response to the wounded in the Civil War. In fact, the Sisters of Charity comprised half of the nuns who ministered to the sick and wounded during the Civil War.

From the roots of the Sisters of Charity of St. Joseph at Emmitsburg, many independent religious communities arose, forming the Sisters of Charity Federation. Among these were the Sisters of Charity of Leavenworth. Their work in healthcare gave rise to SCL Health, an organization of hospitals in Denver, Colorado, that became a founding member of Intermountain Health, one of the largest healthcare mergers (see Chapter 7).

Mother Elizabeth Seton was canonized a saint by Pope Paul VI in 1975, the first person born in America to receive this honor. He praised her, saying, "*May the dynamism and authenticity of her life be an example in our day — and for generations to come — of what women can and must accomplish, in the fulfillment of their role, for the good of humanity.*"[16]

CONCLUSION

The women whose stories are detailed here were extraordinary, but among the religious women of that time they were not unique. We know these women's names, but there were hundreds, even thousands, of others whose names have not been immortalized, but whose commitment to a life of service and poverty, hard work, compassion, and zeal to follow the example of Jesus and the early Church in healing the sick, created the foundations of Catholic healthcare in America.

The meaning of their work gave them incredible resilience and strength to overcome obstacles. They were not building hospitals to enrich themselves or to create healthcare empires. We cannot expect this depth and breadth of commitment and sacrifice from the leaders of Catholic healthcare in our current society, but we should be able to see a strong and true reflection of these values in today's leaders.

CHAPTER 4

The Hierarchy and the Rules

We have been called to form consciences, not replace them.
Pope Francis

Catholicism relies heavily on a clerical hierarchical and a patriarchal structure. The men in positions of authority have long exerted a significant hand in shaping Catholic healthcare from the earliest days of the Church, through the monastic period, and to the present day. These men exerted their influence through prescribed beliefs, teachings, rules, and direct oversight.

THE HIERARCHY

The Catholic hierarchy and lines of authority begin with the pope, extend to the bishops, and then to the priests (Figure 4.1). Fundamental to Catholicism is the belief in a line of spiritual authority that Jesus gave to the apostle Peter and to every pope throughout the millennia. The bishops and archbishops are appointed by the pope and oversee areas of various sizes called dioceses and archdioceses. Priests lead the parishes. The cardinals — the men at Vatican events dressed in red — serve as advisors to the pope, administrators of Vatican areas, and most importantly, are the papal electors.

The pope is designated to be the "Good Shepherd" for the entire Roman Catholic flock. In his role as leader of the world's Catholics, a pope pronounces and endorses dogmas that every practicing Catholic must believe. Despite what many think, there are few Catholic dogmas, and these dogmas are restricted to areas of faith and morals. However, these dogmas do not encompass all that Catholics are asked to believe or all rules by which they are expected to live.

Additional rules emanate from interpretations of the Bible, other teachings, and Tradition. In Catholicism, Tradition with a capital "T" refers to the continuity of the faith handed down by Jesus to the apostles. Tradition with a small "t" refers to matters such as liturgical or devotional activities,

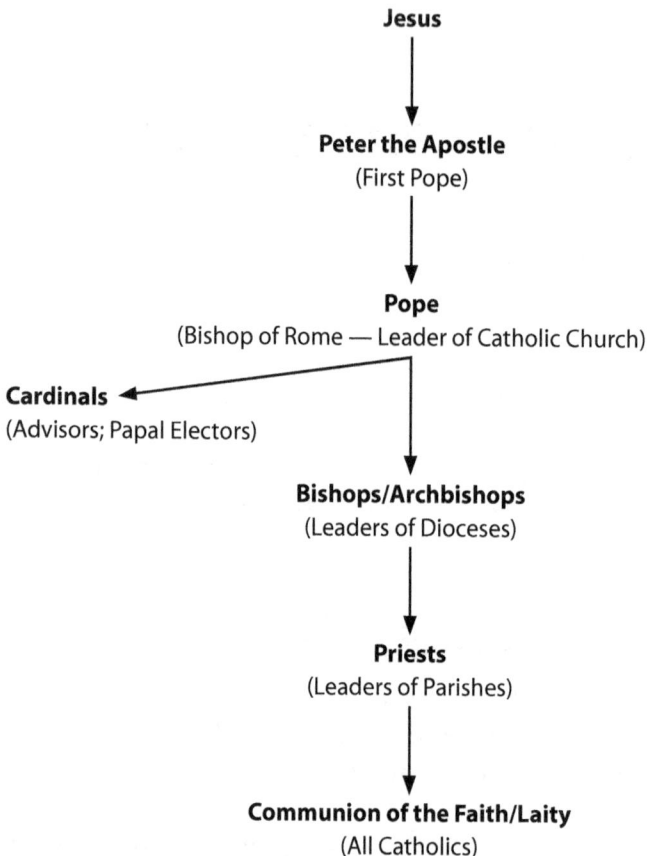

Figure 4.1. Line of Authority and Hierarchy in the Catholic Church

which the popes, bishops, theologians, and other Church leaders develop and promulgate for the entire Church through an interactive dialogue. This dialogue can be a formalized process such as a Council (The Second Vatican Council is an example). Some of the discussions can extend over years, even centuries.

A critical part of the Church's teaching and spiritual direction that the Pope disseminates to the bishops, priests, and all Catholics (some are even directed to all people) are papal letters called encyclicals. Given the significant role that healing played in Jesus' ministry and its centrality in the work of the early Church (see Chapter 1), it is surprising that there is no single encyclical devoted entirely to healing or healthcare. A number of the

TABLE 4.1. Selection of Papal and Bishops Communications Influencing Healthcare

Document(English/Latin)	Writer	Year	Type	Key issue
Of New Things (*Rerum Novarum*)	Pope Leo XIII	1891	Encyclical	Workers' rights
On Human Life (*Humanae Vitae*)	Pope Paul VI	1968	Encyclical	Sexuality/procreation
The Gospel of Life (*Evangelium Vitae*)	Pope John Paul II	1995	Encyclical	Sanctity of life
The Joy of Love (*Amoris Laetitia*)	Pope Francis I	2016	Encyclical	Love in the family
The Good Samaritan (*Samaritanus Bonus*)	Pope Francis I	2020	Letter	End-of-life care
Health and Healthcare	U.S. Bishops	1981	Letter	Health and healthcare
Economic Justice for All	U.S. Bishops	1986	Letter	Social teaching
Doctrinal Note on the Moral Limits to Technological Manipulation of the Human Body	U.S. Bishops	2023	Note	Gender affirming care

encyclicals and other papal documents, however, include important components that apply to healthcare (Table 4.1). The teachings most relevant to healthcare fall into two categories:

- Those that deal specifically with the unique sanctity of human life, sexuality, and procreation.
- Those that address Catholic social mission and obligations.

In the former category, the encyclical that dominates and has had substantial impact on Catholic healthcare is Pope Paul VI's encyclical *Of Human Life, Humanae Vitae,* issued in 1968, which proscribed the use of artificial contraception for married couples.[1] Given that sexual intercourse is allowed only in marriage, it did not address the use of artificial contraception outside of marriage.

At the time this encyclical was issued, some American theologians hoped that contraception would be an issue for individual couples to decide in line with their own conscience. When this was not the outcome, 72 theologians issued a "Statement of Dissent."[2]

More than 50 years later, there is far from unanimity on this position among Catholic theologians, nor is there adherence to this prohibition among many Catholics.[3] In fact, 87% percent of American Catholic women who are at risk for pregnancy use artificial contraception and 98% of Catholic women have used it at some point in their life (see Chapter 5).[4]

Nonetheless, Pope John Paul II and Pope Benedict XVI reaffirmed this prohibition. The writings and teachings of these two popes extended the sanctity of life teaching into proscription against a range of medical interventions including artificial insemination, in vitro fertilization, and euthanasia.[5] Pope Francis has not reversed any of these positions, nor is he likely to do so, but he does appear to have created some space for more dialogue and nuance of these issues.[5,6,7] For example, in his encyclical *The Joy of Love, Amoris Laetitia*, he notes:

> *"...While clearly stating the Church's teaching, pastors are to avoid judgments that do not take into account the complexity of various situations and they are to be attentive ...to how people experience and endure the distress because of their condition."*[8]

He also calls the Church to humility to:

> *"avoid presenting too abstract and almost theological ideal of marriage, far removed from the concrete situations and practical possibilities of real families."*[8]

He emphasizes the role of one's conscience:

> *"We have been called to form consciences, not replace them."*[8]

Of course, this places an obligation on the Church to present the truths that form the correct conscience and on individuals to accept the obligation for forming an enlightened conscience.

Pope Francis' teachings and actions fall heavily into the second category of Catholic beliefs of social mission and obligations. This area is called Catholic Social Teaching, CST. This does and should impact Catholic healthcare. While such teachings clearly began in the Old Testament and flowered with Jesus (see Chapter 1), CST first came to the forefront in contemporary times in 1891 with the publication of Pope Leo XIII's encyclical *Of New Things (Rerum Novarum)*.[9] This was written at a time of great social change and growing wealth disparity across the world — conditions that currently exist in America. The encyclical underscored the right of the Church to speak on societal issues, including private property, workers' rights including the right to organize, and the role of the state and governments.[9]

Since this groundbreaking document, there have been subsequent encyclicals and other documents from seven popes, including several from Pope Francis, that taken together, have given rise to a set of principles that create the core of CST:[10,11]

- The dignity of the human person.
- The dignity of work/priority of labor over capital.
- The person in the community/the common good.
- Human rights/private property/role of government.
- Options for those in poverty/preferential focus on the poor.
- Solidarity/unity of humanity.
- Care for creation.

These principles have direct applicability and relevance to healthcare, including:

- The preferential care of the poor and vulnerable.
- The right to healthcare.
- The evil of excess profit.
- The rights of workers including fair wages and the formation of unions.
- The role of government to intervene to support human needs.
- The judicious use of all resources and care for the environment.[10,11]

In the past, the American bishops strongly supported CST and its intersection with healthcare. This support was captured in two letters: *The Pastoral Letter of the American Catholic Bishops on Health and Healthcare* issued in 1981[12] (copyright USCCB, Washington, DC. All rights reserved. Used by permission) and their letter on *Economic Justice for All* issued in 1986 (copyright USCCB, Washington, DC. All rights reserved. Used by permission)[13] Echoing the messages in the Pope's *Of New Things*, the 1981 document included statements such as:

> "...*the works of justice and mercy are inseparable.*"[12]

> "*Health care is so important for full human dignity and so necessary for the proper development of life that it is a fundamental right of every human being.*"[12]

> "*We believe and hope that American society will move toward the establishment of a national health policy that guarantees adequate health care for all while maintaining a pluralistic approach.*"[12]

> "...inadequate housing, unemployment, lack of education, a polluted environment are frequently the causes of ill health. As church leaders, we will continue to seek social and institutional changes that deal with these underlying problems."[12]

Their letter quotes from a sermon of Pope John Paul II regarding the role of Catholic healthcare's commitment to the poor:

> "*The poor of the United States and the world are your brothers and sisters in Christ. You must never be content to leave them just the crumbs from the feast. You must take of your substance, and not just of your abundance, to help them. Sometimes this will be at great sacrifice and it will demand both courage and imagination. For example, when locating or relocating facilities, leaders in the health apostolate can offer... health care improvement in drastically underserved inner-city and rural areas..."*[12]

The letter also underscores that "*An important and indispensable responsibility of employers is the duty to deal justly with all employees.*"[12]

In 1986, the United States bishops made a forceful endorsement of CST in a pastoral letter, *Economic Justice for All*.[13] This letter contains statements that should be guideposts for Catholic healthcare leaders and a roadmap for overall Catholic advocacy in America:

> "*Economic decisions have human consequences and moral content; they help or hurt people, strengthen or weaken family life, advance or diminish the quality of justice in our land.*"[13]

> "*Every perspective on economic life that is human, moral, and Christian must be shaped by three questions: What does the economy do for people? What does it do to people? And how do people participate in it?... The fundamental moral criterion for all economic decisions, policies, and institutions is this: They must be at the service of all people, especially the poor.*"[13]

> "*...justice requires that the allocation of income, wealth, and power in society be evaluated in light of its effects on persons whose basic material needs are unmet.*"[13]

> "*The concentration of privilege that exists today results far more from institutional relationships that distribute power and wealth inequitably... These institutional patterns must be examined and revised.... For example, a system of taxation based on assessment*

according to ability to pay is a prime necessity for the fulfillment of these social obligations."[13]

"The fulfillment of the basic needs of the poor is of the highest priority. ... policies of private and public bodies ... must all be evaluated by their effects on those who lack the minimum necessities of nutrition, housing, education, and health care. The investment of wealth, talent and human energy should be specially directed to benefit those who are poor or economically insecure."[13]

Some see these as the American bishops' last forceful and far-reaching pastoral letters on CST. When we examine Catholic healthcare today, we should judge it, at least in part, using the principles put forth by the American bishops in the letters on *Health and Health Care* and *Economic Justice for All*.

The inclusion and operational manifestations of the Church teachings on CST and the sanctity of life should both shape Catholic healthcare in America. In fact, when Catholic healthcare began in this country, it seems that CST held the position of prominence and was the primary driver, even though CST was not yet formalized by *Of New Things (Rerum Novarum)* (see Chapter 2). However, in many ways, it appears that the sanctity of life is the predominant force in Catholic healthcare today.[7]

THE LAITY

The Catholic laity should be active and meaningful participants in the life of the Church, but their voices are not always heard or deemed important, correct, or relevant.[14,15] Pope Francis acknowledges this shortcoming and initiated a process to create a venue for all Catholic voices to be heard. In October 2021, he announced October 2023 and October 2024 synods (meetings) of bishops in Rome. During the intervening time, bishops in every diocese in every country are to listen to all the voices via a clear and open process. Pope Francis stated, *"Enabling everyone to participate is an essential ecclesial duty!"*[16]

In announcing this synod, Pope Francis *"...noted that at times there is a type of 'elitism' among the clergy that distances them from the laity, which makes them the 'lord of the house' and not a shepherd."*[16] He envisions something new: *"[W]e need the ever-new breath of God, the Spirit, who sets us free from every form of self-absorption, revives what is moribund, loosens shackles, and spreads joy. There is no need to create another*

Church, but to create a different Church..."[16] Some bishops see this as a great opportunity and others as an impending threat.

THE RULES

While the pope has the ultimate authority within Catholicism, the bishops wield enormous power in their jurisdictions "to set the rules," particularly as they relate to healthcare in the United States. From the bishops' perspectives, the rules accurately reflect papal pronouncements, Catholic theology, and Traditions. This power is clearly demonstrated in the creation, interpretation, and enforcement of the Ethical and Religious Directives for Catholic Health Care Services which have been promulgated by the United States Conference of Catholic Bishops.

Evolution of Ethical and Religious Directives for Catholic Health Care Services (ERDs)

The ERDs have evolved in their content and their operational application over almost 75 years, reflecting in part the changes in Church leadership, science and technology, healthcare institutions, and society (Table 4.2).[7, 17–22]

TABLE 4.2. Evolution of Ethical and Religious Directives for Catholic Health Care Services

Year	Description
1915	Formation of Catholic Hospital Association • Recognized the need for guidelines and standardization.
1921	Written list of prohibited surgical procedures
1948	Publication of *Ethical and Religious Directives for Catholic Hospitals* • Articulated the central role of the bishops in adopting ERDs for their diocese. • Listed procedures that are prohibited, including those in the 1921 list.
1954	Publication of *Code of Ethical Directives* • Chart version of the directives facilitating the posting of the directives.
1956	Publication of Revised Directives • Covered additional areas of care such as psychotherapy. • Included references and an index. • Reaffirmed the role of the bishops in adopting and interpreting the ERDs.
1971	Publication of Revision of *Ethical and Religious Directives for Catholic Health Facilities* • Revision prompted in part by differing interpretation of ERDs in different parts of the United States. • Upcoming potential legalization of abortion. • Covered additional areas such as informed consent, advance directives, cooperation with non-Catholic institutions.

1994	Publication of Revision of *Ethical and Religious Directives for Catholic Health Care Services* • Six sections introduced by theological support for the area. • Added aspects of Catholic Social Teaching including care of the poor. • Covered additional areas of reproductive technologies, surrogate decision-making, advance directives, care of patients in persistent vegetative state, and treatment of rape victims. • Expanded discussion of Catholic and non-Catholic institutional collaboration.
2001	Publication of Revised ERDs • Focus on Catholic and non-Catholic institutional collaboration
2009	Publication of Revised ERDs • Issued in part due to concern about change to lay leadership of Catholic healthcare institutions, changes in healthcare delivery.
2018	Publication of Revised ERDs • Focus on Catholic and non-Catholic institutional relationships. • Administrator conduct regarding procedures at non-Catholic institutions. • Clarified roles of multiple bishops in mergers that cross dioceses and in ongoing assessment of compliance. • Role of Catholics on boards of non-Catholic healthcare institutions.

Information from *Linacre Quarterly*, 1948; *Ethical and Religious Directives for Catholic Health Care Service*, Fifth Edition, Sixth Edition; *Health Progress*, November-December 2019, December 2001; National Health Law Program, January 2019; Salzman, TA and Lawler MG. *Pope Francis and the Transformation of Health Care Ethics*. Washington, DC: Georgetown University Press;2021.

The ERDs dictate what healthcare a Catholic hospital and other parts of the delivery system will and will not provide to patients, independent of individual patient's religious belief, personal conscience, circumstance, or choice; the physician's independent judgement; and the needs and desires of the community in which the institutions are embedded. The ERDs are interpreted and enforced by the local Catholic bishop and not by the hospital board, the community, any governmental agency, or even a diverse group of Catholic scholars.

In their current form, they are a list of "do's and don'ts" with their accompanying moral and theological justification. But that was not their beginning. A Jesuit priest who was a regent of Marquette University and a group of Sisters of St. Joseph of Carondelet who supervised multiple Catholic hospitals wanted assurance that Catholic hospitals were not falling behind in delivering modern healthcare.[2] They were "*concerned that Catholic hospitals become advanced institutions and meet the standards established by accrediting agencies such as the American Medical Association and the American College of Surgeons."*[2]

These concerns gave birth in 1915 to the Catholic Hospital Association (now the Catholic Health Association). The topics at the first meeting of the group reflected these initial concerns: *"The Trend of the Modern Hospital Service, The Significance of Hospital Rating and…The Hospital's Equipment."*[2] The enacted bylaws of the organization reflected both these concerns and their desire to operate in a moral context: *"to advance the general interest of all hospital work, to encourage the spirit of cooperation and mutual helpfulness among hospital workers, to promote, by study, conference, discussion, and publication the thoroughness and correct moral tone and practice of medicine."*[2]

In 1921, these initial efforts to modernize care expanded more into the aspect of standardizing care in keeping with Catholic principles and resulted in a one-page list of "Don'ts/prohibitions issued by the Diocese of Detroit. It focused on surgical procedures, prohibiting destruction of a fetus, and sterilization of men and women.[7,20]

From this beginning, the United States Conference of Catholic Bishops (USCCB) has issued six formal versions of the ERDs (Table 4.2). Over time, these ERDs encompassed addition aspects of healthcare and, more recently, defined how Catholic healthcare institutions can join with non-Catholic entities.

The first complete version of the ERDs was issued in 1948 and started a new era in how Catholic healthcare was delivered within the United States. These initial ERDs enumerated key principles by which Catholic hospitals would operate:

> "Direct killing of… a person is always wrong….
> Every unborn child…[is] a human person… from the moment of conception….
> The unnatural use of the sex faculty (e.g., masturbation) is never permitted….
> Continence …is the only form of birth control that is not in itself morally objectionable"[17]

Application of these principles resulted in a detailed list of prohibited procedures that included direct abortion, surgical procedures to prevent conception, artificial insemination, infertility evaluation that requires semen sample, and euthanasia.[17]

Importantly, the document clarifies the management of care in pregnancy and the acceptability of pain management in the dying. In regard to pregnancy, it states that:

> "*Operations, treatments, and medications during pregnancy which have for their immediate purpose the cure of a proportionately serious pathological condition of the mother are permitted, even though they indirectly cause an abortion, when they cannot be safely postponed until the fetus is viable.*"[17]

The intended reach of the ERDs is articulated, stating:

> "*These directives concern all patients in the hospital regardless of religion and they must be observed by all physicians, nurses, and others who work in the hospital.*"[17]

Significantly, the document affirms the local bishop's role in adopting, interpreting, and applying the ERDs for hospitals in his geographic area.[7,17]

Finally, the document indicates that the Directives will be an evolving effort:

> "*The principles underlying or expressed in this code are not subject to change. But in its applications of principles the code can and should grow and change as theological investigation and the progress of medical science open new problems and throw light on the old ones.*"[17]

The next versions of the ERDs are built on this original document and its principles. The subsequent versions "grow" in scope, but it is less clear that they have changed perspective with expanded theological or medical advances.[2,7] Essentially, every prohibition articulated in the initial version has been maintained and reiterated.

The American bishops strongly supported and welcomed the 1971 version of the ERDs as an approach to reduce the variability of the ERDs' interpretation in different dioceses and because there were concerns about the upcoming Supreme Court ruling on *Roe v Wade*.[7,21]

While the bishops may have been pleased, this edition produced a *"storm of violent criticism."*[21] Some prominent Catholic theologians, most notably Richard A. McCormick, a Jesuit professor, expressed an array of objections detailed in *Not What Catholic Hospitals Ordered*.[23] His objections centered around the theological disagreements within the Church and his assertion that dissenters were not heard; the role of conscience was under emphasized; the implications of implementing the ERDs in a pluralistic, community-based hospital was not considered; and concern that bishops who did not have theological, scientific, or medical training had sole authority.[2,21,23]

McCormick pointed out that Catholic hospitals are supported by public monies and are often the sole community healthcare providers, raising government policy concerns.[21,23] These same issues remain equally relevant today, if not more so, given the expanded reach of Catholic healthcare (see Chapters 5 and 7).

Other revisions ensued in 1994, 2001, 2009, and the most recent Sixth Edition published in 2018 (Table 4.2). While some changes were incorporated, most of McCormick's issues largely remain.

The 1994 edition added at the beginning of the six major divisions, the theological support for the rules that followed. Some attention was accorded to CST. However, some felt that attention should have been given to wages, executive compensation, community needs, and the environment.[21] Most importantly, this edition added instructions on advance directives, use of artificial nutrition and hydration, and application of reproductive technologies that had become available.[7] The most significant change in the Sixth Edition released in 2018 is in Part 6, which concerns collaboration with non-Catholic healthcare entities and adds more constraints to this arrangements (See below).

In June 2023, the United States Conference of Catholic Bishops voted to begin redrafting Part 3 of the Sixth Edition of the ERDs to address the issues delt with in their March 2023 letter *"Doctrinal Note on the Moral Limits to Technological Manipulation of the Human Body,"* prohibiting any medical or surgical gender-affirming intervention[24,25] (see Chapter 5).

An Elucidation of the Sixth Edition of the ERDs

Since the ERDs govern all Catholic hospitals and healthcare institutions in the United States, every entity responsible for healthcare, especially all levels of government, policy makers, insurers, healthcare leaders, and physician organizations, should be aware of the contents of the current ERDs (Table 4.3).

While these individuals and organizations should review the entire document, key portions are listed below. Patients should also have ready access to easily understandable information regarding the ERDs, particularly those components that limit the use of approved medical treatments.

TABLE 4.3. Guide to the Sixth Edition of the ERDs

Part 1 The Social Responsibility of Catholic Health Care Services
Directives 1–9
Key mandates:
- Responsibility to the poor, vulnerable, and marginalized.
- Fair treatment of employees.
- Employee compliance with all ERDs.

Part 2: The Pastoral and Spiritual Responsibility of Catholic Health Care
Directives 10–22
Key Mandates:
- Provision of pastoral care for the religious and spiritual needs of all.
- Provision of sacramental needs of Catholic patients.
- Requirement that the director of pastoral care should be a Catholic and appointed in consultation with the bishop.

Part 3: The Professional-Patient Relationship
Directives 23–37
Key Mandates:
- Provider-patient relationship of trust and confidentiality.
- Commitment to informed consent within ERD constraints.
- Respect for individual's choices only when in compliance with ERDs.
- How advance directives are used.
- Patients' rights and guide for transplantation and medical experimentation.
- When emergency contraception may be used.
- Establishment of ethics committee/consultation.

Part 4 Issues in Care for the Beginning of Life
Directives 38–54
Key Mandates:
- Covers a range of reproductive prohibitions including contraception, assisted reproductive technology, abortion, certain uses of prenatal diagnostics and genetic counseling, and management of some pregnancy complications.

Part 5 Issues in Care for the Seriously Ill and Dying
Directives 55–66
Key Mandates:
- Prohibition of euthanasia.
- Patient should be kept as pain free as possible.
- Patients right to withdrawal of care.
- Requirement for maintenance of food and water even in persistent vegetative state.
- Death determination by a physician or competent medical authority.
- Encouragement for organ donation after death.
- Prohibition of use of tissue obtained from abortion.

(table continues)

TABLE 4.3. *(continued)* Guide to the Sixth Edition of the ERDs

Part 6 Collaborative Arrangements with Other Health Care Organizations and Providers
Directives 67–77
Key Mandates:
• Requirement of bishop's approval of any such arrangement
• Catholic healthcare institutions may not cooperate or have financial benefits with immoral acts as a result of collaboration
• If an entity is under control of Catholic healthcare institution it must abide by the ERDs

Adapted from United States Conference of Catholic Bishops: *Ethical and Religious Directives for Catholic Health Care Services, Sixth Edition.* Washington, DC; 2018

The current version has six major components with a total of 77 directives.[19]

Part 1: The Social Responsibility of Catholic Health Care Services[19]

The introduction to this section emphasizes that the Catholic Church's commitment to healing reflects the belief in the right to life of every human being. It affirms that there is a biblical mandate to the care of the poor, the uninsured, and underinsured. In addition, the Catholic healthcare institutions should contribute to the common good and demonstrate responsible stewardship that reflects equity. Finally, the document makes it clear that Catholic healthcare institutions have the right to refuse to perform procedures they judge morally wrong.

There are nine directives in this section, numbers 1–9.

Directive 3 states:

> "…Catholic healthcare should distinguish itself by service to and advocacy for people whose social condition puts them at the margins and makes them particularly vulnerable to discrimination: the poor, the uninsured and the underinsured; children and the unborn; single parents; the elderly; those with incurable diseases and chemical dependencies; racial minorities; immigrants and refugees."[19]

This seems to require every Catholic healthcare institution to function as a safety-net institution with open doors to the most vulnerable and have in place procedures to prevent discrimination against vulnerable populations.

Directives 5 and 9 require adherence to the ERDs by every employee, including physicians, as a condition of their employment.

Chapter 4: The Hierarchy and the Rules | 63

Part 2: The Pastoral and Spiritual Responsibility of Catholic Health Care[19]

This section underscores Catholic healthcare's commitment to the well-being of the whole person. It deals with the spiritual needs of patients and directs organizations to provide for these needs for all those in their care. Specific mention is made concerning the sacramental needs of Catholic patients.

The section contains 13 directives, numbers 10–22.

Directive 11 states that pastoral service should be available to individuals based on their religious beliefs. Directives 21 and 22 state that the director of pastoral care at a Catholic healthcare institution should be a Catholic and that the bishop must be consulted on the appointment.

Part 3: The Professional-Patient Relationship[19]

This section is critical as it establishes the duties and obligations of healthcare professionals. For physicians, it creates an intersection between the physicians' own consciences, their professed oath, and their employment contracts and practice privileges. These intersecting obligations could, and likely will create ethical and moral dilemmas for them (see Chapter 6).

The perspective section affirms that *"a professional healthcare provider... enter into a relationship (with the patient) which requires... mutual respect, trust, honesty, and appropriate confidentiality."*[19] It further states that the professional care is given *"taking into account the patient's convictions..."*[19]

This statement seems in direct conflict with a critical caveat that follows:

"When the health care professional and the patient use institutional Catholic health care they also accept...the Church's understanding (of) the dignity of the human person.[19] This means that physicians will follow the ERDs as their primary professional code.

The section contains 15 directives, numbers 23–37.

Statements that seem conflicting are in Directives 24, 27, 28, and 36. Directive 24 states that the institution will let the patients know their rights regarding advance directives, but *"will not honor an advance directive contrary to Catholic teaching."*[19] Directive 27 states that patients will receive all information about treatment, but that information must be *"morally legitimate."*[19]

Directive 28 states that patients and surrogates should have information to form their conscience. *"The free and informed health care decision of* the person or the person's surrogate is to be followed so long as it does not contradict Catholic principles."[19] Directive 36 states that "*A female who has been raped should be able to defend herself against potential conception from sexual assault...if ...there is no evidence that conception has occurred.*"[19]

These types of "yes, but" statements align with Catholic teaching, but they likely do not make sense to the average person, including some Catholics. One is left wondering how both parts of such statements can be operationalized.

Part 4: Issues in the Care for the Beginning of Life[19]

This is the section that has sparked and will continue to spark much discussion regarding Catholic hospitals' application of the ERDs.

It affirms "*The Church's ...abiding concern for the sanctity of human life from its very beginning, and with the dignity of marriage and of the marriage act by which human life is transmitted .... Reproductive technologies that substitute for the marriage act are not consistent with human dignity.*"[19]

This section contains 17 directives, numbers 38–54.

Directives 40–42, 45, 47, 48, 50, and 52–54 detail the prohibitions that emanate from the above statement. In the eyes of the Catholic Church, the primary purpose of marriage is procreation, and sexual intercourse in marriage is the only permissible manner of procreation. These deeply held beliefs impact almost every component of reproductive care.

Directives 40 and 41 prohibit heterologous and homologous artificial fertilization. Directive 42 prohibits surrogate motherhood. Directive 45 states unambiguously "*Abortion... is never permitted.*"[19] Additionally, it prohibits cooperation with others who perform abortions.

Directive 48 extends Directive 45 into the terrain of ectopic pregnancies, stating that "*In the case of extrauterine pregnancy, no intervention is morally licit which constitutes direct abortion.*"[19] Directive 47 is important because it does permit lifesaving treatments for women in some circumstances:

"*Operations, treatments, and medications that have as their direct purpose the cure of a proportionately serious pathological condition of a pregnant woman are permitted when they cannot be safely postponed until the unborn child is viable, even if they will result in the death of the unborn child."*[19]

This statement closely mirrors a similar one in the first release of the ERDs in 1948. Directives 50, 52, 53, and 54 contain caveats to permission or prohibition that may lead to lack of clarity for the average person.

Directive 52 states that *"Catholic healthcare institutions may not promote or condone contraceptive practices but should provide...instruction... on responsible parenthood and in methods of natural family planning."*[19] Many would think that spacing or limiting the number of children is a part of responsible parenthood and that responsibility could imply choosing a contraceptive method that is safe, effective, and useable in their circumstance.

Directive 53 prohibits sterilization unless its direct effect is cure of present or serious pathology and a simpler treatment is not possible. An example that would comply with this directive would be surgical intervention for cancer. Directive 50 permits prenatal diagnosis unless it is performed for the possibility of abortion. Directive 54 permits genetic counseling *"in order to promote responsible parenthood"*[19] with the caveat that it must comply with *"the obligations of married couples regarding the transmission of life."*[19]

This section currently does not specifically discuss issues related to homosexuality or gender-affirming treatments or surgeries. However, in June 2023, the bishops issued *Doctrinal Note on the Moral Limits to Technological Manipulation of the Human Body* prohibiting gender-affirming care (See above and Chapter 5).[24]

Part 5: Issues in Care for the Seriously Ill or Dying[19]

Technological and societal trends underscore the need for this section, as they can come into conflict with the Church's position. On one hand, advances in medicine enable physicians and the healthcare system to prolong life beyond what was possible even a decade ago, raising the question of whether the availability of an intervention means that it must be used. On the other hand, in a number of states, the legislative approval of medical aid in dying raises the question of its moral acceptability. The directives chart a middle course on the first question and provide definitive prohibition regarding the second question.

There are 12 directives in this section, numbers 55–66.

Directives 56–59 address the first issue.

Directive 56 states, "*A person has a moral obligation to use ordinary or proportionate means of preserving his or her life. Proportionate means are those that in the judgment of the patient offer reasonable hope of benefit and do not entail an excessive burden or impose excessive expense on the family or community.*"[19] Directive 57 underscores this by permitting a person to forgo extraordinary interventions. Thus, the Church's perspective is that the availability of an intervention does not require its use.

One of the contentious issues in this section is Directive 58, which states, "*...there is an obligation to provide patients with food and water including medically assisted nutrition and hydration for those who cannot take food orally.*"[19] This obligation extends to patients in a persistently vegetative state; the document states that "*such patients can reasonably be expected to live indefinitely....*"[19] There is a "but" stating that this may not be necessary if it will not prolong life or when it is an excessive burden.

Euthanasia is definitively prohibited by Directive 60. Importantly, Directive 61 is equally clear that alleviation of pain is a legitimate goal in care and that medication can be used to accomplish this goal (not the goal of causing death) even if it indirectly hastens the person's death.[19]

Directive 66 appears to be an add-on that does not fit with the theme of care of the dying. It prohibits the use of human tissue from direct abortions being used in research or therapy.[19]

The Good Samaritan (Samaritanus Bonus), a recent letter from the Congregation for the Doctrine of Faith issued with the approval of Pope Francis, further affirms and clarifies the Catholic Church's stance on end-of-life care (see below).[26]

Part 6: Collaborative Arrangements with Other Health Care Organizations and Providers[19]

This section has been expanded in its reach from earlier versions. This undoubtedly reflects the movement of healthcare institutions to mergers and consolidations and to their development of a range of non-hospital-based sites of care. Its purpose is to constrain Catholic hospitals from developing relationships with non-Catholic hospitals that will not follow the ERDs.

> "*When considering collaboration, Catholic health care administrators should seek first to establish arrangements with Catholic institutions or other institutions that operate in conformity with the Church's moral teaching.... they should avoid whenever possible*

engaging in collaborative arrangements that would involve them in contributing to the wrongdoing of other providers."[19]

Collaboration is very broadly defined: acquisition, governance, or management. There are 11 directives in this section.[19]

Directives 70, 73, and 75 detail this overall prohibition. Directive 70 states that

> "Catholic health care organizations are not permitted to engage in immediate material cooperation in actions which are intrinsically immoral, such as abortion, euthanasia, assisted suicide, and direct sterilization.[19]

Directive 73 takes this a step further: "...a Catholic institution must ensure that neither its administrators nor its employees will manage, carry out, assist in carrying out, make its facilities available for, make referrals for, or benefit from the revenue generated by immoral procedures."[19]

Directive 75 prevents a way around these prohibitions by forbidding the creation of another overarching entity that would oversee immoral procedures.

In the past, there were some ways for the non-Catholic hospitals in a merger with a Catholic hospital to continue to care prohibited under the directives. For example, one such approach was to create a "hospital within a hospital" where certain areas of the hospital were incorporated separately.[22] Patients who were to receive certain prohibited services were transferred to this area. Given the expanded constraints, this is no longer permitted.

When one examines the current merged entities that include Catholic and non-Catholic hospitals such as Ascension, Bon Secours Mercy Health, CommonSpirit, Providence, Trinity, and Intermountain Health, it is unclear how they fulfill these directives (see Chapter 7).

This confusion is demonstrated by care provided by the Dignity system, which is not operated under the auspice of the Catholic Church but is part of CommonSpirit, a Catholic healthcare system. Dignity not only refers patients for prohibited procedures, but is proactive in affirming such referrals (see Chapter 7).[27] Directive 73 prohibits physicians from referring patients to a physician at another facility who would perform a prohibited procedure.

As Catholic institutions engage in more mergers and collaborations with non-Catholic hospitals and with other entities, including free-standing emergency departments and urgent care facilities, it will become even more difficult, if not impossible, for patients to know if these facilities are operating under the ERDs.

How these directives are operationalized in the mergers between Catholic and non-Catholic facilities should be of interest to regulators, insurers, communities, providers, and most importantly patients, particularly given the footprint that Catholic healthcare systems now occupy in American healthcare. In fact, these issues are now being raised by some states.[28]

Conclusion of and Reactions to the Directives

The Sixth Edition of the ERDs concludes with an affirmation quoting Jesus' teaching: "*When you hold a banquet invite the poor, the crippled, the lame, the blind....Catholic health care is a response to the challenge of Jesus to go and do likewise.*" [19] This is a noble goal. A question is whether Catholic institutions today seek out and welcome those most in need (see Chapter 8).

Just as there was dissent when the Fourth Edition of the ERDs was released in 1971, there has been discussion and even disagreement among Catholic theologians regarding the Sixth Edition since its initial release in 2009. The areas and reasons for the dissent are provided in detail in *Pope Francis and the Transformation of Health Care Ethics* by Salzman and Lawler, professors of Catholic theology.[7] These concerns include:

- The failure of the ERDs to reflect Pope Francis's broader view for compassion and mercy.
- The lack of dialogue with and inclusion of those who do not agree with the document's drafters nor the inclusion of voices of the entire community of the Church faithful in developing the ERDs.
- The bishops' usurping of the patients' and the health professionals' consciences regarding the care to be provided.
- The failure to integrate CST more fully with sexualteaching.[7]

Salzman and Lawler recommend a revision based on the following words of Pope Francis:

> "We cannot insist only on issues related to abortion, gay marriage and the use of contraceptive methods.... The church's pastoral ministry cannot be obsessed with the transmission of a disjointed multitude of doctrines to be imposed incessantly. We have to find a new balance; otherwise even the moral edifice of the Church [and

Catholic healthcare] *is likely to fall like a house of cards, losing the freshness and fragrance of the Gospel."* [7]

It should be clear that even given this statement, Pope Francis has not reversed the Church's positions on these issues. Moreover, he strongly opposes abortion as part of society's "throw away culture."[29]

Given the USCCB's beliefs and stance on numerous issues related to contraception, abortion, medically assisted death, and gender-affirming procedures and their efforts to have a range of those beliefs not only regulate healthcare choices within Catholic hospitals, but to become law for the country, it seems unlikely that such a revision will occur.

The ERDs and the Papal Encyclicals are critical pillars of the Catholic Church's direction and oversight of Catholic healthcare, but they are not the only source of direction. As noted at the beginning of this chapter, popes and bishops communicate to the body of the Church via formal letters. Two such letters from the American bishops in 1981 and 1986 were discussed above.[12,13] The Papal letter, *The Good Samaritan,* deserves discussion as it augments Part 5 of the ERDs.[26]

The Good Samaritan (Samaritanus Bonus) End-of-Life Care[26]

The advent of medical-aid-in-dying has generated a vigorous response regarding the end-of-life care from the Catholic hierarchy, including Pope Francis. In part in response to the passage of legislation permitting medical aid in dying in a number of countries, the Congregation for the Doctrine of Faith issued a Letter, *The Good Samaritan, Samaritanus Bonus*, with Pope Francis' approval, attempting to further clarify the Catholic Church's stance on end-of-life care.

This letter begins with a question: *"...how do we translate the example of the Good Samaritan [see Chapter 1] into a readiness to accompany those suffering in the terminal stages of their earthly life?"*[26] This letter states emphatically and clearly that *"euthanasia is a crime against human life"*[26] and is *"an intrinsically evil act in every situation or circumstance."*[26] Moreover, any cooperation with this is a grave sin.

The document rejects completely the idea of *"dignified death"* or *"compassionate euthanasia"* to avoid suffering.[26] Part of this rejection is wrapped up in the Catholic belief in the redemptive aspect of suffering, reflecting on the fact that Christ himself suffered and was not spared the anguish that accompanies death. However, the document also makes it quite clear that suffering is not the desired path for patients: *"As the end* draws near, effective pain relief therapy allows the patient to face worsening sickness and death without fear of undergoing intolerable pain."[26]

The document acknowledges that drugs that relieve pain can result in loss of consciousness but that the intent is not to kill the patient, albeit it may speed up the moment of death. It also acknowledges that medical advances can delay natural death, but that these interventions are not only not required when it is clear that the patient is dying, but also that they can interfere with the serenity and dignity of death.

However, the document takes a strong stance on the obligation to provide nutrition:

> "*A fundamental and inescapable principle of the assistance of the critically or terminally ill person is the continuity of care for the essential physiological functions. ….. Nutrition and hydration do not constitute medical therapy but are instead forms of obligatory care.*"[26] There is an important "but." "*When the provision of nutrition and hydration no longer benefits the patient their administration should be suspended.*"[26]

The document also opines on one of the more controversial issues of artificial nutrition: the treatment of patients in a persistently vegetative state. It strongly affirms the continued personhood of these patients:

"*It is always completely false to assume that the vegetative state, in subjects who can breathe autonomously are signs that the patient has ceased to be a human person ..*"[26] It goes on to echo Directive 58 in the ERD that "*The patient in these states has the right to nutrition and hydration, even if administered by artificial means.*"[26] As with the caveats in Directive 58, there is a similar caveat: "*However, in some cases, such measures can become disproportionate, due to ineffectiveness or excessive burden that exceeds any benefits to the patient.*" [26]

Given how carefully worded Papal documents are, it may be noteworthy that this mandate applies to those individuals who can breathe on their own.

CONCLUSION

The Catholic Church's core belief in the unique nature of each person emanates from the teachings found in the Old and New Testament (see Chapter 1). This inherent dignity of every person is a concept that many members of other faith traditions and those not adherent to any religion, value and embrace as foundational to any just and equitable society. So, the question is not the validity or value of this core belief. There is concern, even among Catholic theologians, about the validity of some of the rules that were promulgated from that core belief and that rules that relate to other central beliefs, such as CST, have been omitted.

However, this is not the most pressing issue for our society regarding Catholic healthcare. The most critical issue is that these rules govern the healthcare provided to millions of Americans who are not Catholic, who did not help create these rules, or who do not embrace them as their own.

This imposition of Catholic rules on the healthcare of others appears to conflict with concept of the dignity of every human person, which seems to require acknowledgment and deference to each person's conscience on something as consequential as their own health.

CHAPTER 5

The Impact of the Rules on Patient Care

I ask you is it lawful to do good on the sabbath…?
                                                                 Jesus, Luke 6:9

In a pluralistic society, the enforcement of ERDs by Catholic hospitals and their affiliated entities, particularly as they relate to reproduction, sexuality, and death, should raise issues of public concern regarding:

- The growing reach of Catholic healthcare.
- The potential denial of recognized, effective medical treatments.
- The disproportionate effect on women, including minority women.
- The potential for discrimination based on gender identity.
- The lack of patients' awareness of these rules and the implications for their care.

Each of these issues needs to be examined to get a better understanding of Catholic healthcare in America — the goal of this chapter. Furthermore, given that patients have a legitimate expectation that their care will be based on sound medical practice and not on the physician's or institution's religious beliefs, the chapter examines the level of transparency by Catholic healthcare of their religious structure and their commitment to the enforcement of the ERDs.

CATHOLIC HEALTHCARE'S REACH

Catholic healthcare's importance is a direct result of the large footprint it has on the healthcare terrain. Measures of that footprint include the number of hospitals, the number of hospital beds, and its geographic expanse.

Delineating the exact number of Catholic hospitals is more elusive than one might anticipate. The numbers in available reports vary for multiple reasons. For example, the source of data differs and the timing of the reporting matters, as hospitals are changing hands at a brisk pace, so who owns a hospital in yesterday's report may not be the same owner next week.

Which hospitals are included matters. Do the numbers include pediatric, specialty, psychiatric, and rehabilitation hospitals, or only acute, general hospitals? What is the definition of a "Catholic" hospital? Using different data sets creates the most robust picture of Catholic healthcare. What is quite clear from all these data is that in recent years, the number of Catholic hospitals has increased, and they now represent a sizable portion of the U.S. healthcare sector.

The MergerWatch Project and now Community Catalyst have been monitoring Catholic hospitals for over 20 years. The most recent report from 2020 from Community Catalyst listed several data sources and included all short-term acute, general hospitals with the exception of critical access hospitals, which are small, rural hospitals.[1] A Catholic hospital was considered one that met at least two of the following criteria:

- Member of the Catholic Health Association.
- Member of a Catholic healthcare system.
- Catholic affiliation indicated in public information.
- Inclusion in the Catholic diocese listing.
- Founded by a Catholic entity. [1]

In addition, there was a "Catholic-affiliated" category for hospitals that were in a Catholic system but did not meet two of the above criteria. This very broad definition was purposeful because all of these hospitals may enforce at least some of the ERDs, thereby having an impact on patient care.

With this definition, the study identified 544 Catholic hospitals and 33 Catholic-affiliated hospitals, accounting for 15.8% of the 3,660 short-term acute hospitals.[1] This is a remarkable increase from 449 Catholic hospitals in 2001.[1] This increase occurred as the number of non-Catholic short-term, acute care hospitals decreased by almost 14%.[1]

Another, somewhat smaller estimate of the reach of Catholic healthcare is obtained from the American Hospital Association's (AHA) annual hospital survey in which hospitals provide the information directly.[2] The results of a 2020 survey released in 2021 showed 550 institutions that self-identified as Catholic-operated, acute, general hospitals, representing 12.8% of the 4,288 acute general hospitals in the AHA database (Table 5.1)[2]. Among acute, general hospitals, two groups provide exclusive healthcare to a geographic region: sole community providers and critical access hospitals. These are unique types of hospitals designated by the federal government because they provide the only access to hospital care for Americans living in rural or isolated communities.

TABLE 5.1. Footprint of Catholic Hospitals*

Number of hospitals	550
Number of sole community providers	25
Number of critical access hospitals	133
Number of states with a Catholic hospital	46**/***
Hospitals with more than 300 beds	140
Hospitals with more than 500 beds	29
Total number of Catholic hospital beds	105,578
Number of minor teaching hospitals	281
Number of major teaching hospitals	14
Percent of Catholic hospitals in a healthcare system	96%

*American Hospital Association. Hospital Operational and Demographic Data: FY 2020 AHA Annual Survey Database. www.ahadata.com.
**Data from Solomon T, Uttley L, HasBrouck P, Jung Y. Bigger and Bigger: The Growth of Catholic Health Systems. *Community Catalyst*. February 8, 2020. https://communitycatalyst.org/resource/bigger-and-bigger-the-growth-of-catholic-health-systems.
***The District of Columbia also has Catholic hospitals

Sole community hospitals are designated as such because of the "*hospital's distance in relation to other hospitals, indicating that the facility is the only short-term, acute care hospital serving a community.*"[3] Critical access hospitals are "*[r]ural hospitals maintaining no more than 25 acute care beds...located more than 35 miles, or 15 miles by mountainous terrain or secondary roads, from the nearest hospital.*"[3]

In the AHA hospital survey, 25 Catholic hospitals indicated they were sole community providers (out of 450 sole community providers) and 133 Catholic hospitals indicated they were critical access hospitals (out of 1,353 critical access hospitals).[2,3] These represent 5.6% and 9.8% of these types of hospitals, respectively.

The Catholic hospitals range in size from very small to some of the largest American hospitals. One hundred and sixty hospitals have 50 or fewer beds; these are primarily the sole community providers and the critical access hospitals. One hundred and forty hospitals have 300 beds or more and 29 hospitals have 500 or more beds.

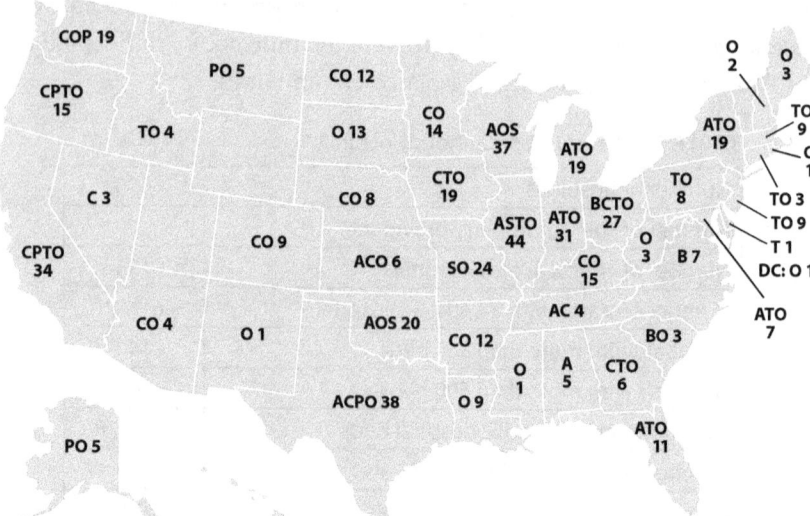

Figure 5.1. Distribution of Catholic Hospitals in the United States
A=Ascension; B=Bon Secours Mercy Health; C=CommonSpirit; P=Providence; S=SSM; T=Trinity; O=Other
Source: Hospital Operational and Demographic Data: FY 2020 AHA Annual Survey Database. Chicago: American Hospital Association, www.ahadata.com

There are a total of 105,578 beds in these Catholic hospitals, representing 14% of all the beds in U.S. acute care general hospitals (Table 5.1).[2] This broad reach is underscored in 2021–2022 reports that four of the ten largest healthcare systems by operating revenue in the United States were Catholic systems.[4]

The Community Catalyst study found that only North Carolina, Utah, Vermont, Wyoming, and Hawaii had no Catholic hospitals (Table 5.2; Figure 5.1).[1,5] With the recent acquisition of five hospitals in Utah by a Colorado Catholic system, there are now only four states with no Catholic hospitals (see Chapter 7). However, there is substantial geographic variation in total number of hospitals, percentage of hospitals that are Catholic, and percent of beds in Catholic facilities (Figure 5.1; Table 5.2).[1]

The percentage of Catholic hospitals ranges from a low of 2% in Mississippi to a high of 43% in Wisconsin. The percentage of beds ranges from a low of 5% in Georgia to 40% or more in Iowa, South Dakota, Wisconsin, Washington, and Alaska (Table 5.2).[1]

The density of Catholic hospitals and of acute care hospital beds in a state does not appear to relate to the percentage of adult Catholics currently residing in that state. For example, in Alaska, 16% of the residents are

TABLE 5.2. Catholic Hospital Staffed Beds, Births, and Adult Catholic Population, by State

	Ranked by Percent of Catholic Beds		
State %	Catholic beds*	% Births*	% Catholics**
AK	46	39	16
WA	41	39	17
WI	40	37	25
SD	40	43	22
IA	40	36	18
NE	38	34	23
CO	38	42	16
MO	37	34	16
OK	32	37	8
OR	30	32	12
IL	28	24	28
OH	27	31	18
KY	27	23	10
IN	26	25	18
MT	25	25	17
MI	23	20	18
ID	23	18	10
ME	23	13	21
AR	22	18	8
NH	20	15	26
LA	20	13	26
KS	19	14	18
CA	17	20	28
ND	16	34	26
AZ	15	19	21
WV	15	20	6
NJ	14	14	34
TX	14	9	23
MA	14	9	34
TN	14	12	6
CT	13	13	33
MN	13	11	22

(table continues)

TABLE 5.2. *(continued)* Catholic Hospital Staffed Beds, Births, and Adult Catholic Population, by State

	Ranked by Percent of Catholic Beds		
State %	Catholic beds*	% Births*	% Catholics**
SC	12	8	10
NY	12	9	31
NV	11	15	25
VA	11	11	12
MD	10	23	15
DE	9	4	22
AL	9	11	7
FL	8	10	21
RI	8	0	42
PA	8	7	24
MS	6	4	4
NM	6	3	34
GA	5	5	9
HI	0	0	20
NC	0	0	9
UT	0	0	5
VT	0	0	22
WY	0	0	14

*Adapted from Solomon T, Uttley L, HasBrouck P, Jung Y. *Bigger and Bigger: The Growth of Catholic Health Systems.* Community Catalyst. Feb 8, 2020. https://communitycatalyst.org/resource/bigger-and-bigger-the-growth-of-catholic-health-systems. With permission.
** Religious Landscape Study: Catholics. *Pew Research Center.* https://www.pewresearch.org/religion/religious-landscape-study/religious-tradition/catholic/. Accessed February 12, 2023. With permission.

Catholic, and 46% of the staffed beds are in Catholic hospitals.[5] In contrast, 22% of Vermont residents are Catholic, but the state has no Catholic hospitals (Table 5.2).[1,5]

Although Catholics represent the second largest religious group in the United States, they constitute only about 21% of the overall population.[5] Therefore, although Catholics may disproportionately use a Catholic hospital, the majority of the population that relies on and uses Catholic healthcare institutions in any state are not Catholics.

Another perspective on the reach of Catholic healthcare is the market share at a local level. One study of 4,450 hospitals in 3,101 counties found that in 35.3% counties, the Catholic hospitals have a high (>20%–< 70%) or dominant (>70%) market share.[6] These counties were estimated to serve 38.7% of women of reproductive age in the United States.[6]

Given the specific and substantial impact of ERDs on reproductive care, it is important to scrutinize not only the percentage of overall beds, but also the percent of births that occur in Catholic hospitals, since the birth of a child is often associated with a range of reproductive advice and care.

As with the variation in the percentage of beds in Catholic facilities, there is wide geographic variation in the percentage of births in Catholic hospitals, with more than 35% of deliveries in Catholic hospitals in South Dakota, Colorado, Washington, Alaska, Oklahoma, Wisconsin, and Iowa and obviously, none occurring in the states with no hospital beds in Catholic facilities (Table 5.2).[1]

Here again, there appears to be no relation to the number of Catholics currently residing in the state, with 25% of the population in Wisconsin and 8% of the population in Oklahoma being Catholic, but more than 35% of the deliveries occurring in Catholic hospitals in both states (Table 5.2).[1,5]

A 2023 study examined the distribution of hospitals with at least 10 deliveries in a year across counties rather than states.[7] The study utilized AHA, Community Catalyst, and Catholic Health Association data in classifying hospitals. There were 2,832 hospitals in 1,618 counties and 14.9% were Catholic.[7] These hospitals delivered 541,626 babies in 2020 — 15.2% of the births.[7] In 181 of the counties, at least 50% of the deliveries were in a Catholic hospital, with all the deliveries occurring in a Catholic hospital in 117 of these counties.[7]

One hundred thirteen of these counties were in areas in which at least one neighboring county also had either no hospitals or no non-Catholic hospitals with at least 10 deliveries, raising concern for access to the full range of maternity and reproductive care, including postpartum contraception, in these counties.[7]

As with the numbers of Catholic hospitals and beds, there are some small differences in the specific volume of care provided in these hospitals based on timing and data sources. What is certain is that Catholic hospitals provide an enormous amount of American healthcare in addition to maternity care (Table 5.3). In 2020, Catholic hospitals had 4,405,674 admissions (14.3% of all acute, general hospital admissions),

472,428 births (13.1% of all births), 94,505,929 outpatient visits (12% of all acute, general hospital outpatient visits) and 17,121,993 emergency department visits (13.8% of all acute, general hospital emergency department visits)(Table 5.3).[2,8] Given the geographic variability in the number of Catholic hospitals in a state, the volume of patient care they provide will vary markedly by state.

TABLE 5.3. Volume of Core Services at Catholic Hospitals and Percent of the Total US Hospital Volume (2020)

Service	Volume	% of Total US Volume
Admissions*	4,405,674	14.3
Births**	472,428	13.1
Outpatient Visits*	94,505,929	12.0
Emergency Dept. Visits*	17,121,993	13.8

*Catholic hospital and total acute general hospital data from AHA data Hospital Operational and Demographic Data: *FY 2020 AHA Annual Survey Database. Chicago: American Hospital Association.* www.ahadata.com
**Catholic hospital births from AHA and total US births from the CDC. Hamilton BE, Martin JA, Osterman MJK. Births: Provisional Data for 2020. *Vital Statistics Rapid Release.* Report No. 012. CDC. May 2021. https://www.cdc.gov/nchs/data/vsrr/vsrr012-508.pdf.

These data underscore the considerable reach of Catholic hospitals. This is an underestimate of the actual impact of Catholic healthcare on patients, since the ERDs are intended to be equally applicable to all Catholic healthcare facilities, including physician practices, urgent care centers, free-standing emergency departments, ambulatory surgery centers, health plans, pharmacies, long-term care centers, and hospices. Furthermore, the prohibitions of some or all of the ERD apply to affiliated non-Catholic partners and their facilities.

How does this considerable reach impact patient care specifically? Although the ERDs have a marked impact on a broad range of care, certain services are most likely to be affected, including contraception, tubal ligation, vasectomy, infertility evaluation and treatments, and end-of-life care (Table 5.4). While the Sixth Edition of the ERDs did not specifically address issues related to gender-identity care, recent communications from the bishops make this an area of emerging concern as well.

CONTRACEPTION

Virtually all sexually active American women have used contraception at some time in their lives.[9] The most commonly used form of contraception is female sterilization by tubal ligations (having the tubes tied), with an

TABLE 5.4. Areas of the ERDs' Impact on Patient Care

Routine contraception
Emergency contraception
Abortion
Management of complications of pregnancy
Management of infertility
Genetic counseling and management of genetic diseases
Management of gender-related care in LGBTQ+ patients
End-of-life care

overall rate of 19% of women, increasing to almost 40% in women aged 40–49.[9] Although it is prohibited by the ERDs (see Chapter 4) 25% of Catholic women use female sterilization for contraception.[10] Presumably, these women had the procedure at a non-Catholic hospital.

The financially and clinically most appropriate time for this procedure, and the standard of care, is at the time of delivery of a child. If a woman wants a tubal ligation and it is not performed then, the procedure requires an admission to another facility and a second procedure, with its accompanying risks, costs, and inconvenience. Neither Catholic nor non-Catholic women giving birth in Catholic facilities can have postpartum tubal ligations.

A 2016 report by the ACLU detailed some cases where this prohibition had a clinically relevant impact, as it did for two women with significant pregnancy risks.[11] Jessica Mann had a pre-existing brain tumor and was pregnant with her third child.[11] Shauna Sharpe had a brain angioma (abnormal blood vessels).[11] Given the medical conditions of these women, the obstetricians caring for them recommended tubal ligation at the time of delivery, but the Catholic hospitals at which the doctors had privileges prohibited this procedure. In these cases, while it may not be ideal, it appears that the patients could choose other physicians at non-Catholic hospitals for their care.

This prohibition becomes a more significant issue for women in rural or remote areas in which there is likely only one source of care. Jennifer Versailles found herself in this situation.[12] She lived in the Colorado mountains and had a scheduled Cesarean section for her upcoming delivery at a Catholic hospital. Although her obstetrician recommended tubal ligation at the time of delivery, this was not permitted by the hospital. The closest other hospitals were 35 and 70 miles away, over mountain roads, which can be impassable at the time of year of the delivery.

Given the dilemma, Versailles obtained legal counsel to address the issue with the hospital, requesting that the hospital allow her doctor to perform the procedure.[12] No details on the outcome of this case could be shared (personal communication with Autumn Katz, senior staff attorney for the Center for Reproductive Rights).

The availability of tubal ligation became an issue of public concern in February 2023 in another rural area of Colorado.[13] The sole community provider in the mountainous southwest part of the state, part of a Catholic system, had not permitted tubal ligations after vaginal deliveries, but the physicians had been performing them at Cesarean section deliveries. With no public notice, the physicians were "re-educated" regarding the prohibitions of ERDs and were no longer able to perform this surgery.[13]

In another case, a legislative aide to a Colorado state representative delivered at a Catholic hospital, expecting to have a postpartum tubal ligation, only to find out that she could not have this procedure.[14] These two examples impacting patient-informed care resulted in legislative action to remedy the situation (See below).

While the focus is most often on surgical sterilization for women, men's reproductive care is also affected by the ERDs; men are unable to obtain a vasectomy in a Catholic hospital.

In addition to prohibiting female and male surgical sterilization, the ERDs prohibit a wide range of contraception. In fact, only natural family planning is allowable.

Although long-acting contraceptive (LARC) methods such as implants and intrauterine devices (IUDs) are approved by the FDA, are highly effective, are frequently covered by insurance, are widely available, and often are the preferred contraception for women, they are prohibited by the ERDs and are not available to women receiving care in a Catholic healthcare facility (see Chapter 4).[15]

However, as with surgical sterilization, there is a disconnect between the rules and what Catholic women do. Twenty-five percent of Catholic women use hormonal methods (birth control pills) and 15% use long-acting contraceptives.[10]

Concerns have been raised that the impact of the ERDs on women's reproductive care may disproportionately affect minority women.[16] Nationally, 53% of births at Catholic hospitals are to women of color, compared to 49% at non-Catholic hospitals.[16] In one study of 33 states and one territory, in 19 of these 34 areas, women of color were more likely to give birth at Catholic hospitals than were white women.[16] For example, in Maryland, 75% of the births at Catholic hospitals were to women of color compared to 48% of the births at non-Catholic hospitals.[16]

On one hand, these data suggest that Catholic hospitals have a more open door and may be more welcoming to women of color — something to be praised. On the other hand, these women may not have available to them the care that they want and from which they would benefit — something not to be desired.

Reproductive care for women living in poverty underscores the complex intersection of religion, government, and politics, particularly as it relates to women whose insurance coverage is Medicaid. Medicaid was the payer for 43% of all deliveries in the United States in 2018.[17] Moreover, in 39 states, more than 35% of all births were covered by Medicaid.[17] It is also the second largest payer of contraceptive services, after private insurance.[18] More than 70% of women whose payer was regular Medicaid or Emergency Medicaid at the time of delivery wanted postpartum contraception and fewer than 5% wanted to use condoms for contraception.[19] None of these would be available to them should they deliver in a Catholic hospital, even though these hospitals are Medicaid providers accepting Medicaid payment.

Are women with Medicaid coverage aware of these constraints before they receive care at a Catholic hospital? At least some are not. Darolyn Lee, a Medicaid patient in Chicago, went to a Catholic hospital that was an in-network provider to have a contraceptive implant replaced.[20] At two clinic visits, the doctors declined to replace the implant with no explanation. The second doctor suggested that she go to the county hospital.[20] Lee subsequently obtained the implant at Planned Parenthood.[20]

In Illinois, all publicly insured individuals must enroll in a managed care plan. Geiseker and colleagues examined the proportion of hospitals with maternity care that were Catholic, other religiously affiliated, or secular that were in the managed care plans in Cook County (Chicago); the racial distribution of patients within the plans; and the impact on family planning in religiously affiliated hospitals.[21]

Five of the seven Medicaid-managed care plans in Cook County had a higher proportion of Catholic hospitals than was the case overall in the county.[21] Eighty-five percent of black and Hispanic women were enrolled in one of these five plans, compared to 75% of white women.[21] There were fewer family planning services provided at the Catholic hospitals and other religious hospitals than at the secular hospitals, even though natural family planning was included in the data.[21] As with the data on births discussed above, this suggests that the religiously affiliated hospitals have a more open door to a minority population, but this is accompanied by limitations in care.

It is not clear how the Centers for Medicare and Medicaid Services (CMS), state Medicaid agencies, Medicaid-managed care plans, or accountable care organizations (ACOs) deal with this issue of contraceptive access in regard to transparency and ease of access to care at other sites.

The ERDs definitely prohibit all contraception but natural family planning, and there are examples of women for whom contraception has been unavailable at Catholic hospitals (see above). Nonetheless, there seems to be a paucity of such examples, given the number of births at Catholic hospitals and the percentage of women who receive care in these hospitals.

There are just a few studies that examine the actual frequency of the Catholic hospitals' prohibitions for a range of contraception. One is the study of Illinois Medicaid-managed care mentioned above. Two survey studies suggest that such prohibitions are not uniform in Catholic healthcare facilities. A small survey study of women in Wisconsin, which has a high percentage of Catholic hospitals, found that only 2% of women had not received the desired contraceptive or fertility care at a Catholic hospital.[22]

A mystery caller study was performed with 144 obstetrics and gynecology clinics listed on Catholic hospital websites. Results revealed differences in the percent of clinic appointments obtained for birth control (type unspecified), copper IUD, and tubal ligation between Catholic-owned clinics and Catholic-affiliated clinics being 84% versus 100% for birth control; 4.4% versus 97% for IUD; and 28.9% versus 71.7% for tubal ligation, respectively.[23] This is a noteworthy difference, as the ERDs would require Catholic-affiliated institutions to follow the prohibitions.

A large study examined the frequency of coding for direct sterilization (tubal ligation) for women at 176 Catholic hospitals.[24] Forty-eight percent of the hospitals performed direct sterilization, suggesting non-uniformity in adhering to the ERDs.[24]

Perhaps the most telling study to examine this issue reported on the frequency of tubal ligations when hospitals changed ownership from non-Catholic to Catholic and vice-versa.[25] When a non-Catholic hospital became Catholic, there was a 31% reduction in tubal ligations.[25] Of note, tubal ligation procedures did not cease, suggesting that hospitals and/or physicians may not strictly follow the ERD prohibitions.[25] There was a smaller increase in tubal ligations when a Catholic hospital became non-Catholic.[25] The smaller change in the latter conversion could reflect that some of these conversions may require maintenance of the ERDs.

This variability of contraception availability, coupled with the lack of hospital transparency, makes it impossible for a patient to know what care will be available. The impact of Catholic healthcare on contraceptive care deserves more detailed study.

Emergency Contraception

Emergency contraception is utilized after unprotected sex and in the instance of rape to prevent pregnancy. In the latter instance, emergency contraception is the standard of care.[26] There were more than 139,380 reported rapes in 2018.[27] Moreover, a CDC study revealed that 14% of teenage girls stated they were forced to have sex.[28] Many of these girls and women may be seen in emergency departments and require timely intervention in order to prevent pregnancy. ERD 36 states that a woman who is the victim of rape should be able to prevent pregnancy due to this assault.[29] Emergency contraception is allowable if pregnancy has not occurred.[29]

Despite the allowability of emergency contraception in the face of rape, it appears to not be uniformly available in Catholic hospitals.[26] A study performed by calls to the emergency departments of a small number of Catholic and non-Catholic urban hospitals revealed mixed operational actions.[26] Twelve of 28 Catholic hospitals and none of 30 non-Catholic hospitals prohibited discussion of emergency contraception.[26] Seventeen of the 28 Catholic hospitals and none of 30 non-Catholic hospitals refused to dispense emergency contraception.[26]

A rape victim — especially a teenage girl — may not have chosen the hospital, known if the hospital is Catholic, or know if the Catholic hospital allows emergency contraception. This places an obligation on the physician and the hospital for transparency and management of the patient within the standard of care, but this appears lacking, as even the discussion of emergency contraception is prohibited by some Catholic facilities.

ABORTION

While maternity care, the availability of post-operative tubal ligation, and the array of contraceptive methods are critically important to a woman's health, it is the issue of abortion that has engendered the most discussion and controversy in regard to Catholic healthcare.

The prohibition of abortion in Catholic healthcare institutions was stated in the first list of "don'ts" written in 1921. It has been restated unequivocally in every version of the ERDs that has been published since the initial version in 1948 and in every papal document that discusses it (see Chapter 4). This prohibition is based on the long and deeply held Catholic tenet that human life begins at the moment of conception.

In recent decades, and more intensely today, it has become clear that the issue of abortion goes well beyond Catholic beliefs and Catholic healthcare. In fact, this broader societal discussion changes abortion from being a solely Catholic healthcare issue to a central issue of legislation and judicial rulings, culminating in the 2022 Supreme Court decision in *Dobbs vs Jackson Women's Health Organization (Dobbs),* which struck down a woman's Constitutional right to abortion in the United States.[30]

This ruling made access to abortion a state issue. By January 2023, 12 states had legislated near-total bans on abortion; two states where there is legal action have no providers performing abortions; four had restrictions based on length of gestation; and three states have bans currently blocked by a court. Three additional states are likely to have legislative actions banning abortions.[31]

In states with near-total bans or restrictions on abortion, providers can face criminal penalties that include fines, loss of license, and jail time.[32] These states are going beyond the Catholic Church's position. Although the Church considers abortion to be a sin, sins are forgivable. While the Church hierarchy in America has been aggressively advocating making abortion illegal, it does not appear to want people to go to jail.

These legislative restrictions in states create geographically different patient access to this care, and have differing implications for Catholic healthcare institutions, depending on the state in which they are located. For example, in South Dakota, there is a near-total ban on abortion, but there are no limitations on abortion in Colorado. Therefore, the 39% of hospitals in South Dakota that are Catholic have the same restrictions as every other hospital in South Dakota. However, in Colorado the 36% of hospitals that are Catholic are operating under different rules than other hospitals, and this may not be understood by patients seeking care.

Additional confusion regarding abortion relates to the fact that 53% of abortions are medication-induced abortions that frequently occur at home.³³ This practice is also becoming the focus of state actions with the banning of prescriptions used in medical abortions. In 2023, Wyoming made it *"illegal to prescribe, dispense, sell or use any drug for the purpose of procuring or performing an abortion"* and attached fines and potential jail time to providers.³⁴

An early 2023 study by the Kaiser Family Foundation found that 49% of women were unsure if medication abortion was legal in their state.³⁵ Moreover, 10% of women living in a state with a complete abortion ban incorrectly thought medication abortion was legal.³⁵ It appears that women are being asked to navigate terrain where even physicians and lawyers may not have clarity.

It is worth noting that abortion was a state issue with regard to Medicaid coverage long before *Dobbs*. A Congressional action known as the Hyde Amendment, adopted in 1977, prohibited the use of federal Medicaid dollars to pay for abortions unless the pregnancy was the result of rape or incest, or the abortion was necessary to save the life of the woman.³⁶ However, states could use their own funds to cover other medically necessary abortions; 17 states do that, paying for all or medically necessary abortions. Despite this inclusion as a Medicaid benefit in these states, it would not be provided at a Catholic hospital.

While the Church's position on abortion and many of the new state laws are unequivocal about the prohibition of abortions, it is an understatement to say there is no uniform agreement among Americans, even among American Catholics, regarding abortion.

An Associated Press poll taken in June 2022, after the release of the draft Supreme Court opinion on *Dobbs*, showed that the opinions of Catholics were similar to the overall population, with 32% of the overall population and 28% of Catholics stating that abortion should be legal in all cases, and 8% and 9% saying it should be illegal in all cases, respectively.³⁷

This poll suggests that Catholics' political party affiliation was more of a determinate of their opinion than their being Catholic. Thirty-nine percent of Catholic Democrats thought abortion should be legal in all cases compared to 10% of Catholic Republicans. Two percent of Catholic Democrats thought it should be illegal in all cases compared to 18% of Catholic Republicans.³⁷

The views on abortion are more nuanced than simply yes or no and are linked to the timing of the procedure. Overall, 67% of those surveyed approved of abortion in the first trimester, while 20% supported legal abortion in the third trimester.[38] This nuanced view on abortion does not appear to factor in either the Church's or some state governments' stance on abortion and, as such, will be a source of disagreement and conflict.

COMPLICATIONS OF PREGNANCY

The ERDs' prohibition of abortion extends beyond elective abortion, impacting the management of two potentially life-threatening complications of pregnancy: miscarriages and ectopic pregnancies. Approximately 1 million women experience a pregnancy loss in the first trimester, and about 10% of confirmed pregnancies result in a miscarriage.[39,40] Eighty percent of patients with first-trimester miscarriages have a completed miscarriage without any intervention within two weeks.[39] However, the other 20% of women may require intervention, which can include continued waiting, medication management with Misoprostol or Mifepristone-Misoprostol, or a procedure.[39] Miscarriage can result in serious hemorrhage or infection; when these complications occur, watchful waiting is not advised.

Given the frequency of miscarriages and their potential complications, how caregivers manage them is critical to women's health. There are reports of women having life-threatening bleeding or infection while experiencing miscarriages because of delayed intervention in Catholic healthcare institutions due to the prohibition against managing the miscarriage with abortion while there are fetal heart tones.[11,41]

An ACLU report describes the experience of a healthcare professional who began experiencing heavy vaginal bleeding at about seven weeks of pregnancy.[11] Realizing that she was having a miscarriage, she went to the Catholic hospital where she worked, as that was the only hospital that was in-network for her insurance coverage. The physician recommended abortion to stop the bleeding. The physician also informed her that the fetus was no longer viable, but since there was still a heartbeat, the procedure could not be performed. The procedure was done seven hours later, by which time she required a blood transfusion.

As with contraception, given the frequency of miscarriage, there seem to be few reports of potential mismanagement and those are case reports of individual patients, not large studies. The study by Hill and colleagues regarding patient care after the conversion of non-Catholic hospitals to Catholic found no increase in the frequency of complications of miscarriages (See above).[25] In fact, there was a decrease in complications for which no explanation was given.[25]

Ectopic pregnancy occurs in 1–2% of pregnancies. In this case, the embryo implants outside the uterus, usually in the fallopian tube. This can result in rupture of the fallopian tube and subsequent severe hemorrhage. Ectopic pregnancy is the leading cause of maternal mortality in the first trimester and accounts for 6% of maternal mortality.[42]

Management can include watchful waiting with the expectation of a spontaneous abortion, medical management, and/or surgical options. Medical management entails the administration of methotrexate, which produces cell death in the embryo and is the most common medical management.

Although it is debated by theologians, surgical removal of the fallopian tube with the embryo might be permissible in a Catholic hospital under the theological principle of double effect.[43,44] This is a somewhat complex but highly relevant Catholic principle which, in the case of ectopic pregnancy, must meet four components:

> "1. *Treatment is directly therapeutic in response to a serious pathology of the mother or the child.*
> 2. *The good effect of curing the disease is intended and the bad effect foreseen but unintended.*
> 3. *The death of the child is not the means by which the good effect is achieved.*
> 4. *The good of curing the disease is proportionate to the risk of the bad effect.*"[43]

However, even using this complex principle, there appears to be no clear guidance on this issue.[43]

The treatment of miscarriages and ectopic pregnancies may be influenced by state laws regarding abortion. A survey of 569 obstetricians in active practice revealed that 44% nationally and 60% of those in states with abortion bans say their professional autonomy has been hindered.[45] Thirty-six percent nationally and 55% in states with bans or limitations say their ability to practice with the standards of care have been impaired.[45] Moreover, 68% stated this has had a negative impact on their management of pregnancy-related emergencies, 64% say it has increased maternal mortality, and 70% state it has exacerbated racial inequities.[45]

These statements are concerning. One has to wonder why obstetricians and gynecologists did not share this same concern about similar limitations in Catholic healthcare institutions, especially in states where a high percentage of deliveries were in Catholic hospitals.

These state actions around miscarriages and ectopic pregnancies produce the same geographic variability as seen with abortion. Here again, the spotlight is being taken off Catholic healthcare as being unique in its approach to care in these circumstances. Thus, this has differing implications for Catholic healthcare institutions based on geography.

Other situations intersect with abortion restrictions as well. One of those is cancer, most commonly breast cancer. About 27,000 women under age 45 are diagnosed with breast cancer each year, and about 4% of those women are pregnant at the time of diagnosis.[46] For some of these women, optimal treatment of the cancer is not feasible due to pregnancy.[46] Although some of these patients are receiving care in Catholic hospitals, there do not appear to be reported cases where this was a dilemma for these patients.

Since the recent *Dobbs* decision and subsequent state bans on abortion, numerous articles in the medical literature have raised serious questions about how this will affect women's health in the circumstances noted above. In fact, almost the entire November 1, 2022, issue of the *Journal of the American Medical Association* was devoted to this concern.

Moreover, 75 medical societies, including the AMA, issued a joint statement declaring that the *Dobbs* decision is a threat to a person's well-being and health, as well as patient-centered and evidence-based care.[47] Given that abortion has been a clear prohibition in Catholic hospitals at least since 1948, it is puzzling as to why there was no such organized pushback in response to the prohibition in Catholic hospitals.

- Perhaps these groups were more willing to oppose state laws than Church laws.
- Perhaps it is the fact that a state law affects every hospital.
- Perhaps these groups did not appreciate the extent of the reach of Catholic healthcare.

Whatever the reasons, it appears the issue is not addressed, as none of the many articles discuss the specific impact of the Catholic healthcare's prohibition of abortion on people's health.

INFERTILITY

While controlling pregnancy numbers and spacing is a concern of many couples, infertility is the concern of others. About 10% of couples have not been able to have a child after two years of being sexually active.[48] The impact of the ERDs on this area of reproductive care has had less focus.

A standard infertility evaluation includes the evaluation of both partners, since infertility is related to the male partner one-third of the time, the female partner one-third of the time, and both partners or an undetermined cause one-third of the time.[48] The ERDs create a barrier to pursuing the male partner's role in infertility, as masturbation to obtain a semen specimen is prohibited. Some obstetricians have suggested it may be permissible to obtain a semen specimen with intercourse using a condom with a pinhole that could permit conception to occur. However, infertility evaluations in a Catholic system may be incomplete.

Management of infertility is an area of medicine that has seen considerable technological advances over recent decades. However, most of these advances are prohibited by the ERDs.

Directive 38 puts considerable restriction on infertility care, allowing only "… *assistance that does not separate the unitive and procreative ends of the act, and does not substitute for the marital act itself.*"[29] There are specific prohibitions against heterologous (Directive 40) or homologous (Directive 41) artificial insemination.[29] Directive 39 prohibits in vitro fertilization (IVF) since with this technology there are embryos that cannot be implanted and may be destroyed.[29]

The issue of future infertility arises in individuals with cancer who are receiving chemotherapeutic agents that will likely cause infertility. These individuals may wish to bank sperm or embryos. The procedures needed to do this are not permitted in Catholic facilities. Just as the issue of abortion has moved from an issue for Catholic healthcare to the broader society, it is likely that the status of embryos and IVF will move to a broader debate.

GENETIC DISORDERS

Issues arise in couples seeking genetic assessment for a range of clinical concerns including "a *heritable condition in one (or both) of the couple, a history of infertility or recurrent pregnancy loss, a family history of one or more possibly heritable conditions, a couple who is from a population group with a high frequency of certain genetic diseases, and couples who are blood relatives.*"[49]

When transmission of a genetic disease is being considered, the American College of Obstetricians and Gynecologists recommends pre-conception screening that would enable a couple to consider any pregnancy, screening of embryos, or other reproductive options such as using donor gametes, deciding not to have children, and adoption.[49]

The post-conception option of abortion in the face of a serious genetic defect is clearly not an option in a Catholic hospital. While genetic testing is permitted in Catholic institutions, it cannot be used as a reason to utilize any of the prohibited reproductive options; it can only be used to prepare a couple for having a child with a serious disease or disorder.

LGBTQ+ CARE

Gender-related care extends beyond women's reproductive care to include providing care for LGBTQ+ patients. There are two aspects to the care of this group of patients: routine, regular healthcare, and gender-affirming care. Care for conditions and diseases that any person could have should not be in question. However, that does not mean that such patients would not face discrimination in a Catholic healthcare setting. In fact, it appears that some level of discrimination is supported.

A National Catholic Bioethics Center publication states: "*...no Catholic health care organization should require its personnel to carry out, promote, refer for, or otherwise cooperate formally in procedures involved in gender transitioning, especially surgical or hormonal interventions; require the use of pronouns or sex-specific identifiers that are explicitly contrary to a person's biological sex; or otherwise require the affirmation of a false sexual identity for any persons who are or who are planning on transitioning.*"[50]

Other Catholic bioethics publications go further: "*Furthermore, Catholic facilities should not implement gender-affirming protocols for example, allowing patients claiming transgender beliefs to access opposite-sex bathrooms or requiring all staff to undergo sensitivity training that would pressure them into using patients' preferred gender pronouns.*"[51]

To address this issue of discrimination of LGBTQ+ patients in all hospitals, the Human Rights Campaign developed a Health Equity Index to "*promote equitable and inclusive care for LGBTQ+ patients and their families.*"[52] This Index measured the presence of several major policies, including patient non-discrimination and training, patient services and support, and employee benefits and policies.[52]

The organization examined 2,200 hospitals, including the 906 hospitals that participated in a survey.[52] The Veterans Health Administration had the largest number of participating hospitals.[52] One hundred nine academic medical centers and 65 faith-based facilities, of which 23 were Catholic hospitals, participated in the survey (personal communication to Tari Hanneman, Human Rights Campaign).[52]

Of the Catholic hospitals, 15 were members of the Dignity System in California and two were part of academic medical systems in Ohio and Pennsylvania (personal communication, Tari Hanneman, Human Rights Campaign). Eighty-two percent of all institutions participating in the survey earned a designation of Leader or Top Performing, indicating the adoption of anti-discrimination policies.[52]

While this does not imply that the other facilities not participating in the survey, both Catholic and non-Catholic, were engaged in discrimination in care, it does suggest they were not focusing on non-discrimination of this population of patients.

The areas most in question in the care of this group of patients are the treatments and procedures specifically targeted to alter the sex at birth to the identified gender of the individual. A publication expressing Catholic bioethics has unequivocally declared such treatments immoral: "*First, no Catholic provider should directly carry out gender transitioning ..., Catholic physicians and organizations should not authorize the maintenance of cross-sex hormones or other transitioning regimens... no referrals should be made directing or recommending that patients undergo gender-transitioning intervention.*"[51]

This prohibition of any gender-altering intervention was further affirmed in March 2023 in a formal statement of the American bishops, *Doctrinal Note on the Moral Limits to Technological Manipulation of the Human Body.*[53] In that document, the bishops state:

> "*Catholic health care services must not perform interventions, whether surgical or chemical, that aim to transform the sexual characteristics of a human body into those of the opposite sex or take part in the development of such procedures. They must employ all appropriate resources to mitigate the suffering of those who struggle with gender incongruence, but the means used must respect the fundamental order of the human body.*"[33]

Using this as a stepping-off point, the bishops voted unanimously at their June 2023 meeting to begin a process to revise the ERDs to address the issue of transgender care.[54]

How the bishop's Doctrinal Note, and Directive 73 of the ERDs, which governs affiliations and referrals (see Chapter 4), are operationalized across the terrain of Catholic healthcare is unclear. This is exemplified by the practice within the Dignity system, which is not operated under the auspice of the Catholic Church but is part of CommonSpirit, a Catholic healthcare system.⁵⁵ Dignity facilities not only refer patients for prohibited procedures, but also are proactive in affirming such referrals (see Chapter 4):

> "*Our network of care includes, but is not limited to, offerings such as hormone therapy, psychological services, mastectomy, breast augmentation, orchiectomy, and hysterectomy, although not all services are available at all facilities.*
>
> *When a service is not available at a given location, care is transitioned to a provider within reasonable driving distance that offers the desired service. .*"⁵⁵

In May 2023, the Lepanto Institute for the Restoration of All Things in Christ issued "*an investigative report into the largest Catholic health system in the United States and its performance and funding of transgender surgeries and therapies, abortions, and its prescribing and provision of contraception,*" calling out Dignity/CommonSpirit.⁵⁶ This may have contributed to the bishops decision to revise the ERDs to address transgender care.

A Catholic ethics publication goes even further in the prohibition of gender-affirming care, stating that such treatments should not be included in the coverage in any of their insurance plans: "*Catholic organizations that offer their own insurance products or that are self-insured should categorically exclude sex reassignment surgeries and all other forms of gender transitioning from their coverage*"⁵¹

There is both questioning and dissent within the Catholic religious community on this position. Rev. Charles Bouchard, senior director of theology at the Catholic Health Association, noted in response to the bishops' plan to revise the ERDs, "*The biggest issue is our understanding of human sexuality. Will we into the future continue to see human sexuality as what we call binary, male and female, or are there shades in between?*"⁵⁴

A coalition representing 6,000 vowed religious individuals issued a letter in March 2023 stating, "*As members of the body of Christ, we cannot be whole without full inclusion of transgender, non-binary, and gender-expansive individuals.*"⁵⁷ In addition, the Sisters of Mercy released a statement on the Trans Day of Visibility, saying, "*We are learning to appreciate dimensions of human dignity we did not know existed. We promote education that expands our social, scientific, pastoral and religious understandings of all persons as created in the image and likeness of the Divine.*"⁵⁸

One teacher of Christian ethics at a Catholic College commented that the bishops' statement lacked humility "*in the face of the stories that transgender people tell about who they are as well as the face of emerging scientific and medical discussions around gender identity."*[59] A professor of moral theology at another Catholic college criticized the bishops' statement as cherry-picking from papal documents to support their perspective, stating, *"Transgender health care presents the Catholic moral tradition with questions that are very complex. Two of the most significant popes cited in the clarification consistently reminded us that the person is far more than their body alone. Even as the USCCB has chosen to follow a narrow tradition that inconsistently places the good of persons behind the functionality of their body parts, the moral tradition itself continues to offer many more expansive interpretive possibilities."*[60]

Pope Francis has not changed the Church's teaching on homosexuality, but as is his overall Catholic understanding of inclusivity and mercy, he has condemned laws criminalizing homosexuality as unjust.[61] In June 2023, in a statement on the upcoming worldwide Synod (meeting), he asked for "radical inclusion" of the LGBTQ+ community.[62]

LGBTQ+ care is not only an area of religious discussion, but also new terrain for legal battles. In 2019, a patient in California sued Dignity for refusing to perform a hysterectomy for a transgender male. The Court of Appeals upheld the patient's right. Dignity had already transferred the patient to another facility for the procedure.[63] In 2023, a similar case occurred at a Catholic hospital in Maryland, with the judge awarding a summary judgment to the patient.[64] These will most certainly not be the last cases regarding a range of gender-affirming care.

While there are no specific gender-affirming care requirements in the Medicaid program, this may become an area of legal question, since the Medicaid program has a requirement of providing comparable services to eligible groups.[65] Just as there is variation in Medicaid coverage of abortion, there is also variation in coverage of gender-affirming care.[65] Moreover, as with abortion, this will have differing impact for Catholic institutions, depending on whether the availability of their services aligns with the state's coverage.

In the recurring theme of state laws mirroring Catholic beliefs and prohibitions, as of March 2023, 18 states have passed laws or policies that restrict gender-affirming care for minors.[66]

END-OF-LIFE CARE

While the beginning of life holds great importance, if for no other reason than the continuation of the species, the end of life also holds importance as a transition point from one generation to the next, and for many religions, the transition from this existence to another. Thus, in many ages, religions, and cultures, each of these moments holds a prominence worthy of rituals and rules.

The Catholic Church is no exception. The beginning and the end of life also share some definitional issues, albeit there is more debate about the timing of the beginning of life than the end of life. As discussed above, for the Catholic Church, life begins at conception, and death is defined as natural death. This commitment to natural death clearly impacts end-of-life care.

But as they say, "Death is not what it used to be."[67] When we die, what we die from, and where we die have changed dramatically since the last century. At the beginning of the 1900s, death often occurred in infancy, making old age and its attendant maladies somewhat uncommon. In that pre-antibiotic, pre-vaccine time, communicable diseases, including tuberculosis, influenza, and diphtheria, were the leading causes of death, followed by heart disease, stroke, and malignancy.[67] The infectious diseases had little effective treatment, let alone cures. The other causes of death, including cancer and cardiovascular disease, were beyond the reach of medical therapeutics.

But public health and therapeutic advances have changed all that. Before the COVID pandemic in 2018, six of the top 10 causes of death were diseases such as heart disease which have long courses in comparison to many infectious diseases.[68] This, along with other forces, have changed the places where we die, which greatly impacts how we die.

Early in the last century, most people died at home. Even by 1949, only about 50% of people died in an institution, and for a majority of them it was a hospital.[67] As hospital services and medical technologies expanded, more people were in the hospital at the time of death, perhaps to avail themselves of advances in care.

By 1980, 74% of deaths were in a hospital.[67] Dying in a hospital created the opportunity and momentum for more interventions to prolong life, or in many cases to stretch out dying. However, in recent years this trend toward death in a hospital has reversed, no doubt reflecting a changing view of death itself. In 2017, for the first time, the percentage of deaths at home exceeded those occurring in hospitals: 30.7% at home and 29.8% in hospitals.[69] Today's newspaper obituaries often recount, "She died peacefully at home surrounded by her family."

Added to this mix of options for the place of death was the establishment of hospices for end-of-life care. Although the first hospice was established in 1974, the percentage of deaths occurring in hospices did not substantially increase until the mid-2000s, rising from 0.2% of deaths in 2003 to 8.3% in 2017.[69] Dying at home or dying in hospice seems to be in accord with the concept of natural death.

These changes in age of death, causes of death, and place of death have both clarified and complicated Catholic healthcare at the end of life. First, what natural death is may not be as obvious as it was in the last century. The Oxford Dictionary defines natural as *"existing in nature, not made or caused by humans."* That covers a great deal of terrain including, on the face of it, any medical intervention. In fact, what a natural death was 100 years or even 50 years ago likely meant something different to most people than what it does now. For our great-grandparents or even our grandparents, when a serious illness struck, there was little recourse from "natural death."

The incredible advances that have moved average life expectancy from about 50 years in 1900 to 77.3 years in 2020 may well have blurred our view of natural death.[67,70] One might legitimately ask, "Does cardiac resuscitation prevent natural death?" "Does mechanical ventilation prevent natural death?" "Does cancer chemotherapy prevent natural death?" "Does tube-feeding or intravenous nutrition prevent natural death in a person in a vegetative state?"

One could generate hundreds of variations on these questions and every doctor and certainly every patient and their families will have different questions and different answers.

But from the perspective of Catholic healthcare, it is the Church's answer that matters. Some of its answers are included in Part 5 of the ERDs and the papal letter *Samaritanus Bonus,* discussed in Chapter 4. Both of these documents are clear that the availability of technologies that prolong life does not mean that they are required when they are not beneficial or when they are excessively burdensome or interfere with the serenity of death. The one exception to this is the mandate for supplying nutrition, even if it is by artificial means, and even for those in a vegetative state (see Chapter 4).[71]

While there is some current discussion about changing the definition of brain death,[72] the Church continues to rely on the standard definition: *"The determination of death should be made by a physician or competent medical authority in accordance with responsible and commonly accepted scientific criteria."*[29]

While there is substantial information in medical literature and the press regarding Catholic hospitals' enforcement of the ERDs concerning multiple aspects of reproductive care, there is relatively little on the impact on end-of-life care for specific patients. It would be interesting to know if end-of-life interventions are more intense or more common in Catholic hospitals than in other hospitals. For example, are there more admissions in the last month of life, are there a greater number of ICU days, more procedures and other tests, fewer DNR orders in terminally ill patients, or are there fewer patients with advanced directives in Catholic hospitals than in other hospitals?

One of the most consequential and controversial aspects of dying today is the possibility for a person to choose how and when to die in the face of a terminal disease. These choices are enabled by the medical-aid-in-dying laws enacted in 10 states and the District of Columbia.[73] The Church unequivocally prohibits this, as is clearly stated in the ERDs and in *The Good Samaritan (Samaritanus Bonus)*.[71]

In Colorado, a legal challenge was mounted relating to a Catholic healthcare institution terminating a physician for writing prescriptions for life-ending medications that were not for use in the hospital.[74] Under Colorado law, a physician was permitted to do this regardless of the employer's stance on the issue. The Catholic system has asked that the case be moved to federal court. The twist in this case is that the system is arguing against an individual physician's right to act in line with her religious beliefs. Usually, this argument has been used to shield physicians from acting *against* their beliefs.[75] As of February 2023, the case had yet to be decided.

TRANSPARENCY

Although the limitations of services are of major concern, equally important is patients' and the community's awareness, or more accurately the lack of awareness, of these limitations. Twenty to 30% of Catholic hospitals do not identify their religious affiliation, and for those that do, that designation may not be particularly easy to find.[76-77] Of the websites of 652 Catholic hospitals, more than two-thirds required more than three clicks from the home page to find out if they were Catholic.[76] Another study found comparable results, with only 79% of Catholic hospitals listing their religious identity if one looked at the home page, "About Us," and/or the Mission statement locations on the website.[78] How many patients will do that amount of searching, especially since patients may not even be aware that the religious affiliation of the hospital can impact their care?

Seventy-one percent of surveyed patients did not consider religious affiliation when selecting a hospital.[79] The Catholic ownership and direction of the hospital may not have seemed important because patients do not understand the implications. In fact, 71% of individuals believe that their own healthcare choices should be the deciding factor in care, not the dictates of the religious belief of the facility.[79]

If patients do persist in finding out if a hospital is Catholic, what would knowing the Catholic identity tell them about the limitations of care? Examination of 646 websites of Catholic hospitals showed that 76% did not cite the ERDs on their website and only 15% provided a link to the ERDs.[78] However, even for the few that link to the ERDs, that may not be sufficient to inform patients of unavailable care, as these are not presented in a way that enables the average patient to understand care limitations.

Moreover, among the 494 Catholic hospitals with no mention of ERDs, only 4% provided information on specific care restrictions and/or end-of-life care restrictions.[78] In one study, fewer than 3% of the websites *"contained an easily found list of services not offered for religious reasons and all of them were in Washington state which requires such information …."*[76] Even with Washington state's requirement that hospitals post their policies on reproductive and end-of-life care, only six of the 20 Catholic hospitals in the state did so in an easily accessible place.[76]

Why would the ERDs and the specific care limitations for a hospital be so hard to find? This is an especially interesting question, given that by standing by their Catholic moral principles, these hospitals intended to be an example for society. One wonders if the lack of transparency relates to not deterring patients from using the hospital, thereby enabling the hospital to maintain its market share and revenue.

This lack of transparency on care restrictions is relevant, as most patients are not aware of what Catholic hospital affiliation dictates for provisions of care. Using two hypothetical hospitals, subjects were asked to identify if a hospital was Catholic or non-religious by its name (Saint's John vs. Metropolitan) and then, if identified as Catholic or non-religious, to indicate if they thought they would be able to receive any one of nine possible treatments: birth control pills, tubal ligation, D&C for miscarriage, abortion for fetal indications, abortion for life-threatening pregnancy, abortion for personal reasons, in vitro fertilization, delivery, and natural family planning.[80]

If they identified a hospital as Catholic, over 60% of the respondents thought they could get a prescription for birth control pills and a tubal ligation; 71% thought they could get a D&C for a miscarriage; and over 40% thought they could get an abortion for a life-threatening pregnancy, and could have in vitro fertilization.[80] Only 12% thought they could get an abortion for personal reasons, but 27% thought they could get an abortion for fetal indications.[80] Even 30% percent of Catholic women who attended service monthly thought they would be able to have an abortion for serious fetal indications.[80]

Another survey revealed that almost 70% of individuals did not anticipate a difference in healthcare based on the hospital being Catholic.[81]

All patients receiving care in any healthcare facility are given and must sign a consent form for treatment, except in an emergency situation in which they are unable to sign. Therefore, the content of the consent forms is a critical component of a healthcare facility's transparency. There appears to be no systematic study of hospital consent forms regarding this issue. Apparently, a high level of transparency is so unusual that a Texas newspaper reported that St. Luke's Hospital, a Catholic hospital in Texas, actually listed in detail all procedure and referral limitations that it followed based on religious beliefs.[82]

These concerns regarding lack of transparency are magnified in two specific groups of hospitals---sole community providers and critical access hospitals. In 2020, 25 of the 450 (5.6%) sole community provider hospitals were Catholic hospitals (see above). In my review of these twenty-five websites in 2023, only two indicated on the hospital's website landing page that it was a Catholic hospital; one each indicated that the hospital was Catholic in the website's Mission, Values, or History section. Four of these also had a saint's name. One might infer that another eight were religiously affiliated, but not necessarily Catholic since they had a saint's name. Three hospital websites indicated they followed the ERDs. Twenty-three of the 25 sole community providers were members of a system, of which 14 indicated they were Catholic. One other strongly implied that. Four of these systems' websites indicated they followed the ERDs and had a link to them.

This recently became a public issue in Colorado when a sole community healthcare provider changed its policy on postpartum tubal ligations with no public announcement (See above).[13] In 2020, 132 of the 1,353 critical access hospitals (CAH) were Catholic facilities (see above). Although there is no data for CAHs regarding transparency, there is no reason to believe that it would differ from that of the sole community providers or from Catholic hospitals overall.

When a leader of the Catholic Health Association was asked about not listing excluded services or not having certain services, he replied that no hospital leads with what they do not have, and many hospitals do not offer every service.[76] Of course, that's correct. However, secular hospitals are not excluding services based on religious beliefs. Therefore, the exclusion does not have the same potential to create conflict between the organization's religious beliefs and those of the patient. Moreover, services excluded by secular hospitals are not necessarily services that patients expect to be provided, nor would these hospitals prevent a referral of a patient to another hospital for the services they do not provide.

The first point is highly relevant given that one of the most frequent reasons for hospital admission is childbirth and, hence, women would expect that services related to pregnancy and childbirth would be provided. Therefore, this lack of transparency appears to differ in important and relevant ways from what might be appropriate in other circumstances.

Since the government is now requiring hospitals to be transparent about pricing, it seems obvious that it should require transparency about service restrictions, since this can be a life-or-death issue, not a pocketbook issue. In fact, this is now starting to happen. The 2023 Colorado legislature passed a bill labeled the Patients' Right to Know Act.[82] Starting in 2024, healthcare facilities must inform patients, through the informed consent process, of the services that the healthcare facility refuses to provide for non-medical reasons.[83]

While the discussion in this chapter has focused on hospitals, healthcare is provided in many venues, including free-standing surgical and other care centers, emergency departments, urgent care centers, outpatient facilities, and by telemedicine, and is directed by health plans and ACOs, including those owned or affiliated with a Catholic healthcare organization. There is little information on their operationalizing of ERDs.

For most patients, whether the hospital accepts their insurance, the reputation of the hospital, and the recommendations from others dictate their choice of facility.[79] Since having care where insurance will apply is critical to patients, it would seem that insurance companies also have an obligation to clearly indicate if hospitals that are in-network have care restrictions related to their religious affiliation. There does not appear to be any data on insurance companies' policies on this issue.

CONCLUSION

Catholic healthcare institutions are a major component of American healthcare. They provide a significant amount of care to patients in rural and urban America, often disproportionately serving minority populations. But there is a caveat to this care: The ERDS prohibit important components of standard medical care in these institutions.

The ERDs were promulgated by the American bishops to ensure that every Catholic healthcare institution operated within the framework of Catholic moral theology and religious belief. While the motivation was rooted in genuine belief and moral convictions, these rules are far-reaching and impact the healthcare and patient autonomy of many millions of non-Catholics as well as Catholic patients.

There is also a lack of transparency by these institutions, resulting in patients being unaware that the religious beliefs of their healthcare institution dictate their care, often in critical ways. The Church and society need to wrestle with the dilemma of institutions providing much-needed care, but also withholding other care from patients without regard to their wishes.

CHAPTER 6

Fulfilling Oaths and Following Conscience

May I never see in the patient anything but a fellow creature in pain.
Maimonides

The ability of Catholic hospitals and physicians to withhold some medically accepted care from patients based on their own religious and moral beliefs is made possible by numerous protections of religious freedoms. However, patients look to their physicians as trusted partners in their care who will act solely in their best interest and include them in care decisions. These two realities come into conflict at both the individual and societal levels, and therefore, deserve discussion. This chapter examines:

- The training of future physicians in Catholic healthcare.
- The responsibilities of physicians to their patients as dictated by their professional oaths.
- The intersection of these responsibilities with Catholic institutions' mandate that physicians follow the ERDs.
- The breadth of the legal protection for Catholic hospitals and their physicians in the exercise of their religious beliefs.

IMPACT ON PHYSICIANS

Trainees

Patient care within the U.S. health system is directed by licensed professionals — frequently physicians. Often, they oversee and contribute to the training of medical students and physicians in their post-graduate years as interns, residents, and fellows. This training occurs in a hospital setting, including Catholic hospitals.

Two hundred eighty-one of the 550 Catholic hospitals are minor teaching hospitals and 14 are major teaching hospitals.[1] These institutions assume responsibility for providing all the post-graduate training needed for a person to be a competent physician. However, in Catholic hospitals, trainees are not exposed to any of the services prohibited by the ERDs, nor do they engage in shared decision making with their patients for these services. They may face moral dilemmas in withholding certain types of care. To obtain the required experience, trainees are often sent to other institutions for some periods of time.

The Accreditation Council for Graduate Medical Education (ACGME), the body that accredits all training programs in the United States, does not specifically identify which programs are in Catholic hospitals (personal communication Kathleen Quinn-Leering and John Combes ACGME).[2] However, the ACGME affirms that all the training programs in a specific discipline, including obstetrics and gynecology, have the same requirements.

The review committees that grant accreditation review the programs annually, examining case logs of the residents' procedures, resident and faculty annual surveys, annual program updates, and percent of residents passing the board examinations, which has a threshold of 80% (personal communication Kathleen Quinn-leering and John Combes, ACGME).

Despite this extensive information about the training program and trainees, it is not clear that adequate clinical training occurs. A small interview study of obstetricians and gynecologists practicing in secular institutions who had completed residency at a Catholic hospital one to five years previously revealed that *"none of the interviewees felt their program provided sufficient off-site training in all areas of family planning to compensate for the lack of these elements in their regular curriculum and experiences."*[3] They also reported that when they entered practice, they needed a variety of strategies to compensate for this gap.[3]

In the 1990s, (personal communication, John Combes, ACGME) the ACGME took legal action against a program at a Catholic hospital for failure to comply with the requirements, but there have been no similar actions since then. However, other actions may have been taken against training programs.

Physicians

There is a belief that goes back to ancient times that physicians have unique responsibilities in relation to the care of patients. Since Hippocrates in the 5th century BCE, physicians have been expected to take an oath professing their responsibilities to the patients they serve. This first oath began with the commitment to do no harm and to maintain confidentiality.[4] In the 12th century, Maimonides, a renowned Jewish rabbi, philosopher, and teacher, expanded the obligations in the oath accredited to him to include commitment to truth and warnings against avarice and pursuit of glory:

> "The eternal providence has appointed me to watch over the life and health of Thy creatures. May the love for my art actuate me at all times; may neither avarice nor miserliness, nor thirst for glory or for a great reputation engage my mind; for the enemies of truth and philanthropy could easily deceive me and make me forgetful of my lofty aim of doing good to Thy children."[5]

Centuries later in England in 1803, Thomas Percival, a physician and philosopher, offered further guidance on physicians' behavior. He focused more on a physician's conduct in relationship to a hospital, than on philosophical or moral principles. In 1847, the American Medical Association adapted his document into a code of medical ethics.[6] However, like Maimonides, the current AMA Code of Medical Ethics places a moral responsibility on physicians:

> "The practice of medicine, and its embodiment in the clinical encounter between a patient and a physician, is fundamentally a moral activity that arises from the imperative to care for patients and to alleviate suffering. The relationship between a patient and a physician is based on trust, which gives rise to **physicians' ethical responsibility to place patients' welfare above the physician's own self-interest or obligations to others**, to use sound medical judgment on patients' behalf, and to advocate for their patients' welfare."[7] [Author's bold] (Used with permission of the American Medical Association. ©American Medical Association 2023. All rights reserved.)

This statement seems quite clear on where the physician's responsibility lies, but it is followed by a caveat related to the physician's own conscience:

> "Preserving opportunity for physicians to act (or to refrain from acting) in accordance with the dictates of conscience in their professional practice is important for preserving the integrity of the medical profession as well as the integrity of the individual physician, on which patients and the public rely. Thus physicians should have

considerable latitude to practice in accord with well-considered, deeply held beliefs that are central to their self-identities."[7] (Used with permission of the American Medical Association. ©American Medical Association 2023. All rights reserved.)

However, Stahl and Emanuel contend that in choosing the profession of medicine, one has committed to putting the patient above all else:

"By entering a health profession, the person assumes a professional obligation to place the well-being and the rights of patients at the center of professional practice.... In a professional context personal religious convictions are secondary."[8]

While the AMA Code of Medical Ethics seems to be slightly at odds with this statement, the code's support for personal conscience has its caveats:

"Physicians' freedom to act according to conscience is not unlimited....

In following conscience, physicians should:

Thoughtfully consider whether and how significantly an action (or declining to act) will undermine the physician's personal integrity, create emotional or moral distress for the physician, or compromise the physician's ability to provide care for the individual and other patients.

Before entering into a patient-physician relationship, make clear any specific interventions or services the physician cannot in good conscience provide because they are contrary to the physician's deeply held personal beliefs, focusing on interventions or services a patient might otherwise reasonably expect the practice to offer.

Take care that their actions do not discriminate against or unduly burden individual patients or populations of patients and do not adversely affect patient or public trust...

Uphold standards of informed consent and inform the patient about all relevant options for treatment, including options to which the physician morally objects.

In general, physicians should refer a patient to another physician or institution to provide treatment the physician declines to offer."[7] (Used with permission of the American Medical Association. ©American Medical Association 2023. All rights reserved.)

The American Society of Obstetrics and Gynecology agrees with the need for physicians to inform potential patients of their moral objection to certain standard procedures and to refer patients who need or want these procedures.[9] A survey of 1,144 physicians from a range of specialties revealed that 71% believe that when a patient requests a legal medical procedure that the physician has a religious objection to performing, the physician has a moral obligation to refer the patient to a physician who does not have that objection.[10]

The belief that physicians have an obligation to refer a patient in this situation was held by 82% of low religiosity (their assessment) and 56% of those with high religiosity — 55% of Catholic physicians, 65% of Protestant physicians, and 80% of Jewish physicians.[10]

The ERDs' Part 3 focuses on the professional-patient relationship, acknowledging that "*A person in need of health care and the professional health care provider who accepts that person as a patient enter into a relationship that requires among other things, mutual respect, trust, honesty, and appropriate confidentiality.*"[11]

Yet, the ERDs require physicians to follow the ERDs, which appear to prevent the discussions and referrals of prohibited procedures (See above and Chapter 4).

These statements appear to be in direct conflict with each other and in conflict with the AMA code, professional society recommendations, and the general opinions of physicians. At least one Catholic healthcare system, SSM, does not permit referrals for prohibited procedures, (personal communication Patrick Kampert SSM) (see Chapter 7).

It is not only Catholic institutions that place constraints on physician's autonomy with employment contracts. Most physicians are employees of a healthcare entity, and those entities have employment contracts. These requirements are not as extensive in their reach, and they focus primarily on financial issues. However, some of these requirements may violate the conscience of individual physicians and their professional code, particularly regarding preferential service to insured over uninsured or other vulnerable patients.

Nothing in the AMA code states that employment contracts supersede a physician's moral obligation to the patient. In fact, "…the *AMA Code of Medical Ethics obligates the physician — regardless of setting or institution — to uphold the ethical norms of the profession, including patient self-determination, which may be in conflict with their own cultural, religious or philosophical beliefs" (Personal communication, Jack Resnick, Jr. MD, President AMA, November 28, 2022).*

"So," one must ask, "how does the Catholic institutional employment requirement to adhere to the ERDs intersect with the physician's professed oath and the physician's own conscience?" "What ethical principle would allow an employment contract to supersede a physician's oath and her/his own conscience?" "How does the sacred covenant of physician with a patient, which is a mutual commitment, become a one-way transactional relationship?"

Catholic hospitals' websites do not list what percentage of the physician staff are Catholic nor do they identify which of the physicians are Catholic. One would not expect that they would. However, given that only 21% of the population is Catholic, it is highly unlikely that all, or even a majority, of the physician staff are Catholics. In fact, of the over 1 million active physicians in the United States in 2022, only about 980 physicians were members of the Catholic Medical Association (personal communication, Elizabeth Griffin, Catholic Medical Association).[12]

Thus, the question of conscience could easily arise with those non-Catholic physicians who practice at Catholic hospitals. In fact, given the Catholic laity's view on many issues, some Catholic physicians may not agree with the directives in the ERD and have similar dilemmas of conscience. These dilemmas would be particularly likely among the obstetricians who feel that prohibitions on specific treatment negatively impact their autonomy and patient care (see Chapter 5).

An example of this dilemma is described by a physician who was prohibited from performing a tubal ligation at the time of a patient's cesarean section, requiring the patient to have an additional procedure:

> "…[I]f you're doing a c-section on somebody that wants a tubal and has had six other previous c-sections and… if I tie her tubes I'm going to get kicked off the staff. And I just don't think that's right but … instead of benefiting my patients, I benefit myself and don't do the tubal and stay on staff. So that's difficult sometimes."[13]

There is another twist for physicians who are not employees of a Catholic healthcare system but have hospital privileges through medical staff appointment. In that case, it seems they would be governed by the medical staff bylaws.

I am unaware of any study of the medical staff bylaws of Catholic hospitals or of their inclusion of a set of religious behaviors as criteria for the granting of hospital privileges. However, examination of the medical staff bylaws that were available on the internet for at least one hospital in each of the CommonSpirit, Providence, Ascension, and Trinity health systems, and another Catholic hospital not a member of one of the large systems, revealed that each required that a medical staff member abide by the ERDs.

The most surprising of these bylaws was Ascension's, which stated: "*Should there be any conflict between any provisions of the applicable Code of Ethics (*which for physicians was the AMA Code of Medical Ethics [author]) *and the Ethical and Religious Directives, the latter shall prevail.*"[14]

The specific prohibition of abortion and some gender-affirming care by states now presents physicians in these states with moral and ethical dilemmas similar to those of physicians in Catholic hospitals. A flurry of articles in medical journals appeared after the *Dobbs* decision and the subsequent states' abortion prohibitions regarding the impact on the patient-physician relationship.[15]

Moreover, a question has been raised that if these care limitations harm patients and are unjust, is civil disobedience to these restrictive laws warranted.[16] One wonders why these questions were not asked before or even now in relation to Catholic healthcare.

The moral dilemma that physicians face regarding care, particularly in regard to abortion for medical complications, is further complicated by the legal and career-ending risks to physicians created by states that have imposed criminal violations for performing or facilitating abortion.[17]

How did we get from physicians' primary responsibility being to the patient, to their right to exercise their own conscious, to religious institutions dictating the bounds of the doctor-patient relationship and the provision of care? The journey was much less about a debate within the profession or a debate by ethicists, and much more about the actions by politicians, lawyers, and judges.

CATHOLIC HEALTHCARE, ERDS, AND THE LAW

A series of legal and political actions have enabled the American Catholic hierarchy to create and enforce the ERDs in Catholic healthcare (Table 6.1). This path starts with the First Amendment of the U.S. Constitution. The enforcement of one set of religious beliefs by a government or ruler is probably as old as religion and government. The more diverse a society is,

TABLE 6.1. Evolution of Laws on the Exercise of Conscience

Action	Year	Key Elements
First Amendment	1791	Free exercise of religion. No government-established religion
Church Amendment	1973	Exempts federally funded individuals and facilities from requirement to perform abortions or sterilization if they have a moral objection. Nondiscrimination in employment or promotion of physician or other personnel if they perform or would not perform abortion or sterilization.
National Research Service Award Act	1974	Exempts individuals from participating in federally funded research if they have a moral objection.
Religious Freedom Restoration Act	1993	Forbids any government entity from burdening a person's exercise of religion without compelling government interest.
Coats-Snowe Amendment	1996	Forbids the withholding of accreditation of physician training programs due to failure to provide abortion training; allows students to abstain from abortion training.
Balanced Budget Act	1997	Permits insurance companies to deny coverage, payment, or referrals on basis of conscience.
Weldon Amendment	2005	Forbids funding of institution that discriminates against those who refuse to perform, offer referrals to, or cover abortions. Insurers are not required to cover these services

the more intrusive or restrictive the enforced rules are, and the larger the percentage of the population impacted, the greater the concerns regarding governmental laws based on one religion.

Our Founding Fathers recognized the dilemma of this intersection of religion and government and tried to thread that needle in the creation of the First Amendment:

> *"Congress shall make no law respecting an establishment of religion, or prohibiting the free exercise thereof; or abridging the freedom of speech, or of the press; or the right of the people peaceably to assemble, and to petition the Government for a redress of grievances."*[18]

The first phrase of this amendment constitutes the Establishment Clause; the second phrase is the Free Exercise Clause. This amendment was intended to give Americans important and highly valued protections, but the Establishment Clause and the Free Exercise Clause have and will continue to come into conflict. Religious leaders, politicians, lawyers, and judges, have and will continue to debate the boundaries of both clauses of the First Amendment protections.

Catholic hospitals' ability to impose the ERDs and other rules on physicians and other providers, Catholic and non-Catholic, and on their many patients, Catholic and non-Catholic, has been permitted under the Free Exercise part of the First Amendment and its interpretations and extensions.

Does this violate the Establishment Clause by giving one religion governmental blessing? Given the concern about government overreach that was represented by the Establishment Clause, one has to wonder if the Founding Fathers intended that institutions whose primary activity is not the practice of religion, but rather the provision of healthcare to the population, largely with taxpayer dollars, should be able to use the Free Exercise Clause to establish what care is given or not given.

As states enact laws that mirror the ERDs, particularly around reproductive care, the debate about where the line between the Establishment Clause and the Free Exercise Clause falls will go beyond Catholic hospitals and their care. Some would say that the line is crossed when harm comes to others:

> *"Religious freedom means the right to our beliefs. That right is fundamental and must be vigorously defended. But religious freedom does not give us the right to impose our views on others, including discriminating against or otherwise harming them."*[19]

So, as we examine the laws that extend the Free Exercise Clause, it seems wise to use that lens: Does the protection result in harm to some individuals?

There has been a march to extend the Free Exercise Clause reach for individuals and to have it apply to a broad range of institutions with the passage of numerous laws and rules: The Church Amendments, the National Research Service Award Act, the Religious Freedom Restoration Act, the Coats-Snowe Amendment, the Balanced Budget Act of 1997, the Weldon Amendment, and the "Conscience Rules" (Table 6.1).

The Church Amendments were enacted as part of the Public Health Act in 1973, shortly after the *Roe v Wade* decision.[20] These amendments protect federally funded healthcare personnel who will not perform procedures such as abortion, sterilization, or medical aid-in-dying because they object on moral or religious grounds.[20] What is almost never mentioned but deserves to be underscored is that the Church Amendments also prohibit discrimination in employment, promotion, or termination of healthcare personnel who perform these procedures.[20]

While these amendments were likely a response to *Roe v Wade*, their justification came from a very unusual place: the conscientious objection to the military draft that became a major issue during the Vietnam War.[8] Stahl and Emanual analyze why the objection to the draft and a physician's objection to care differ in important ways.[8] Key among these differences are:

- Conscription is not a choice, but being a healthcare provider is a choice, including the choice to practice in disciplines in which there likely will be procedures that the provider finds morally objectionable.
- The sincerity of the objection to military service is evaluated through external assessment, but there is no such process for physicians or others to assess how deeply held physicians' objections are.
- The military conscientious objector must provide alternate service, but this is not an obligation of the physicians or others who claim a conscientious objection to performing some procedures.[8]

Others have pointed out another clear difference when the conscientious objector is a physician or a healthcare facility:

> *"Religious exemptions can trigger or unleash consequences for third persons. It is therefore impossible to characterize conscientious objections as a right that affects solely those who exercise it."*[19]

A year after the Church Amendments, the National Research Service Award Act permitted individuals to refuse to participate in research to which they have religious or moral objections.[21] The Religious Freedom Restoration Act of 1993 prohibited any agency, department, or official of the United States or state *"from substantially burdening a person's exercise of religion even if the burden results from a rule of general applicability, except that the government may burden a person's exercise of religion only if it demonstrates that application of the burden to the person: (1) furthers a compelling governmental interest; and (2) is the least restrictive means of furthering that compelling governmental interest."*[22]

This appears to apply only to individuals and not institutions. One could reasonably ask if guaranteeing the right of everyone to access medically indicated/appropriate care is a compelling governmental interest.

A series of other Congressional amendments and administrative actions extended the Church Amendments. The Coats-Snowe Amendment was passed in 1996 in response to a new Accreditation Council for Graduate Medical Education requirement that residencies in obstetrics and gynecology include training in abortion procedures. This amendment underscored that the right of conscience is not only a power of an individual, but also of an organization. The amendment prevented withholding a program's accreditation based solely on the failure to provide this training and exempted institutions and individuals from this training.[23] This has obvious implications for the training of physicians (see above).

The massive omnibus Balance Budget Act of 1997 permits insurance companies to deny coverage and referrals based on conviction. This is a further extension of the concept of conscience to a major institutional component of American healthcare.[8,24]

In 2005, the Weldon Amendment broadened the reach of conscience and attached a big stick to these rules by forbidding funding of any institution or healthcare entity *"that discriminates against those who refuse to perform, offer referrals to, or cover abortion services."*[8,25] This broad language enabled insurance companies who were considered healthcare entities to exclude coverage for abortion.

The so-called "Conscience Rules" are not a Congressional action, but rather rulings by the Department of Health and Human Services. They address the protection of persons and institutions on matters concerning religious beliefs and moral convictions. These rules demonstrate the political influence and, therefore, the volatility that molds these rules. In 2009, the Bush administration declared that a person was *"protected from mandatory participation in treatments or research that was contrary to their religious beliefs or moral conviction."*[8,26]

The 2019 "Conscience Rule" was a far-reaching rule in terms of the number of statutes included entities, individuals, and services covered; and enforcement of the rules.[26,28] The covered entities included not only institutions providing services, but also those paying for services. All employees working in a healthcare institution were covered, including clerical staff who could refuse to provide services with which they had moral objections. Strong enforcement components were added.[27] Physicians, lawyers, and ethicists voiced concerns about this rule on many grounds:

- It covered individuals who had no overarching professional obligations to the patients.

- Physician's primary duty is to the patients.
- It distorts the balance between the physician's exercise of conscience and the patient's right to care.
- It ascribes to institutions a conscience, which is a characteristic ascribed to individuals.
- There is a distinction between the freedom to believe and the freedom to act on that belief. In the latter instance, the potential to harm others cannot be ignored.[28–31]

The rule reflects how controversial this terrain is, as it was instituted during President Trump's administration, but President Biden's administration planned to rescind it.[32]

The First Amendment Free Exercise Clause, Congressional actions, and administrative rules regarding the reach of religious freedom form the legal umbrella under which Catholic healthcare has been able to limit the provision of certain medically indicated and/or acceptable treatments or procedures to the many non-Catholics who rely on their institutions for healthcare. However, even with these legal umbrellas, there are some questions.

Prior to the Church Amendments in 1973, it is not clear what gave the Catholic healthcare institutions the legal umbrella to refuse the care prohibited in the 1948 ERDs and continuing until 1973. Was anyone asking that question? Although none of these amendments establish a line that cannot be crossed regarding the provision of care, it seems possible that Catholic healthcare institutions may have gone beyond the limit in refusing to provide contraception to patients. While there are protections for refusing surgical sterilization and paying for contraceptive coverage, the amendments do not appear to include the right to refuse to counsel patients about or dispense contraceptives. There are challenges which have recently occurred relating to gender-affirming surgery. This suggests that the broad religious exemptions for institutions may indeed have limitations (See above).

Another critical intersection of the law and ERDs relates to the Emergency Medical Treatment & Labor Act (EMTALA).[33] The EMTALA statute, enacted in 1986, created a federal obligation, tied to receipt of Medicare funds, to ensure that patients, specifically pregnant women, have access to emergency care, including screening and stabilizing treatment.[33] Stabilization requires that appropriate treatments be provided to prevent the patient's clinical deterioration. Patients can be transferred to another facility if the initial hospital does not have the capability for the needed treatment or if the patient requests a transfer.[33]

The potential for conflict between the ERDs and EMTALA arises when a woman is experiencing a miscarriage or an ectopic pregnancy. This can precipitate a medical emergency in which abortion could be medically indicated. This intersection is now occurring not only in Catholic hospitals, but also in hospitals in those states that have banned or severely restricted abortion.

Following the *Dobbs* decision, HHS issued guidance stating, *"If a physician believes that a pregnant patient presenting at an emergency department is experiencing an emergency medical condition as defined by EMTALA, and that abortion is the stabilizing treatment necessary to resolve that condition, the physician must provide that treatment. When a state law prohibits abortion and does not include an exception for the life of the pregnant person — or draws the exception more narrowly than EMTALA's emergency medical condition definition — that state law is preempted."*[34]

This warning was followed a number of months later with a Centers for Medicare and Medicaid Services' investigation of two hospitals, one in Kansas and one in Missouri, neither of which were Catholic, that concluded that they were in violation of EMTALA for failing to provide abortions to women suffering from miscarriage.[35] As states restrict abortion and even apply criminal consequences to those who perform abortions, there will likely be debate about what constitutes a medical emergency in a pregnancy.[17, 36,37]

One wonders why this guidance and such investigations did not occur years earlier in regard to the ERDs' prohibition of abortion. Why is this only now an issue when the state bans are coming into play?

CONCLUSION

The ERDs can create moral dilemmas for the physicians who practice in Catholic hospitals and other healthcare facilities, with tension between their professional oaths, their own conscience, and their employment contracts. One could, and should, ask how one religion can dictate the healthcare of so many others who do not share those beliefs. Ironically, this has been enabled by the First Amendment of the Constitution and subsequent laws, regulations, and judicial rulings that uphold the freedom to exercise religious beliefs, as individuals and as institutions, while impacting the freedom of others in something as basic as their health and life.

The intersection of this freedom with the First Amendment's prohibition of government-sanctioned religion will continue to be examined, not only as it relates to Catholic healthcare and its prohibitions, but also regarding states' laws that impact the provision of healthcare. Where the boundary lies between these two pillars of freedom does and will continue to profoundly affect the delivery of healthcare in America, impacting the health of many millions of Americans, especially those with limited choice of a provider. As Americans we must continue to discuss and examine this boundary.

CHAPTER 7

The Landscape of Catholic Healthcare

You must...not allow the spirit of the world that makes gods out of power, riches, and pleasure make you forget that you have been created for greater things.
                                                                    Mother Teresa

A series of strong forces reshaped American hospitals over the last century, transforming American healthcare from a small cottage industry of local providers into a complex, powerful, and profitable industry. Understanding this transformation is essential to understanding Catholic healthcare in America today. Many of those forces have impacted all hospitals, but some have had a particular effect on Catholic hospitals, and a few have been unique to them. These forces can be divided into financial and non-financial ones (Table 7.1).

FINANCIAL FORCES

New payment methods for care and construction emerged beginning in the 1930s and have continued to the present time. These methods moved all hospitals from modest billing of individuals for care and charitable funding for care of the poor, core operations, and capital acquisition and construction, to billing third-party payers and structured capital financing.

The first of these major financial changes was the development of third-party payments for care by commercial insurance products starting in the 1930s. In part, this was an effort to preserve hospital income in the face of the Depression. Blue Cross, Blue Shield, and the Kaiser Foundation Health Plan were operational by the end of the 1930s, but by 1940, only 9% of Americans had some private health insurance.[1] However, this changed rapidly during the war years, and by 1950, 50% of Americans had some private health insurance. By 1970, over 75% of people had some private coverage.[1]

TABLE 7.1. Forces of Change on Catholic Healthcare

Financial Forces	Start Date
Commercial Insurance	1930s
Hill-Burton Program for construction	1946
Medicare and Medicaid	1965
Disproportionate Share Program (DSH)	1980–1981
Children's Health Insurance Plan (CHIP)	1997
Affordable Care Act (ACA)	2010
HHS Provider Relief Fund	2021
Mergers and consolidations	2000
Non-financial Forces	
Decrease in the number of women religious	1963
Legalization of contraception	1965;1972
Constitutional right to abortion (*Roe v Wade*)	1973
Reversal of right to abortion (*Dobbs*)	2022
Assisted reproductive technology	1978
Medical Aid-in-Dying laws	1997
Conscience laws and rules	1973

Health insurance created a new revenue source for hospitals beyond what patients could pay themselves, and it escalated competition among hospitals to capture these patients and their revenue streams — efforts still very much in play today.

A major transition from relying on philanthropy for capital acquisition and construction to a specific funding source was the passage of the Hill-Burton Program in 1946.[2] This was an important infrastructure bill for hospitals and other healthcare facilities. From 1947 to 1971, $28 billion poured in for the construction and modernization of healthcare infrastructure, facilitating the addition of more than 70,000 hospital beds.[3]

Catholic hospitals were one of the recipients of this government money, with 80% of them receiving Hill-Burton funds.[4] This bill was notable not only for its impact on hospital expansion, but also as the first action to tie the receipt of government support to an obligation to provide community benefit, which in this case was the provision of free or subsidized care to some patients.[5]

As important as the Hill-Burton Act was in expanding the footprint of American hospitals and facilitating their journey to becoming a powerful economic force, an even more profound change was produced by the enactment of Medicare and Medicaid in 1965, which helped pay for the care of many of the patients occupying these beds. Over time, these two programs expanded both the eligible individuals and the services that were covered.

Although the uninsured who relied on hospital charity care remained, those numbers dropped with new government coverage. As of March 2023, Medicare covered 65,748,297 individuals[6] and Medicaid covered 86,714,574 individuals.[7] The federal expenditures for these programs in 2021 were $900.8 billion and $734 billion, respectively.[8] Thus, with these two programs, the financial underpinnings of the healthcare system and the federal government's role as an insurer changed significantly.

Closely linked to Medicare, and most particularly to Medicaid, was the creation of the federal government's Disproportionate Share Program (DSH), which Congress established as part of the Boren Amendment to the 1980 and 1981 Omnibus Budget Reconciliation Act.[9] The DSH program instructed states to consider a hospital's portion of Medicaid and uninsured patients in establishing hospital payments. These payments help defray the cost of this care.[11]

States slowly adopted these special payments, and by 1990, the total Medicaid DSH payment was $1.4 billion.[9] Through various legislative actions and a variety of mechanisms to enhance the Medicaid DSH federal match, in FY 2020, the total Medicaid DSH payments grew tremendously, totaling $19.5 billion ($8.2 billion in state funds and $11.3 billion in federal funds).[10]

Although the federal government has established DSH caps and some basic rules, states create formulas to determine specific DSH payments to individual hospitals. Thus, the amount of DSH payments a hospital is entitled to receive, if any, is determined in large part by the state in which it is located.[10] Fifty-six percent of short-term, acute care hospitals, 53% of not-for-profit hospitals, and 67% of 417 non-critical access Catholic hospitals reported receiving DSH payments.[11-13] These payments decrease a hospital's expenditure on the care of uninsured and underinsured patients.

While children do not represent a large portion of hospital admissions, expenses, or revenue, the enactment of the Children's Health Insurance Plan (CHIP) in 1997 offers free or low-cost coverage to children in families (some states cover pregnant women) whose incomes, while low, exceed the threshold for Medicaid coverage. This added one more piece to the federal funding streams available to hospitals.[14]

One of the recent impactful financial forces was the passage of the Affordable Care Act (ACA) in 2010. This is estimated to have given healthcare coverage to 35 million Americans, 21 million of whom have coverage from Medicaid in those states that opted for expansion of the program.[15] This legislation drastically decreased the percentage of uninsured individuals from 16% pre-ACA to 8% in 2022.[16]

While the ACA reduced the number of uninsured that hospitals cared for, including those cared for in Catholic hospitals, it also generated unique issues for Catholic healthcare regarding mandated covered services that were prohibited by the ERDs.

The COVID pandemic created enormous clinical and financial challenges for all hospitals; not all hospitals bore these burdens equally.[17,18] The federal government's COVID Relief Fund helped hospitals weather these challenges by infusing $178 billion to hospitals, albeit not equally.[18] Some institutions struggled with patient volume and revenue, while some achieved significant profits during this time.[18] Two of the largest Catholic systems, CommonSpirit and Ascension, received more than $1 billion each.[18]

The large infusions of federal dollars via these and other funding programs helped patients access care and also enabled healthcare to become exceedingly profitable and powerful. Catholic healthcare systems, along with every other hospital, reaped the financial benefits.

Another financial force, somewhat independent of the infusion of dollars that significantly changed the healthcare landscape, was the merger, acquisition, and consolidation of hospitals with each other (horizontal consolidation) and with other components of the delivery system (vertical consolidation).[19–21] The rationale for these consolidation efforts was better coordination of services across facilities and regions, improvement in quality by sharing best practices, economies of scale, and ultimately decreased cost and increased profits.

According to one report, 10% of hospitals were in systems in 1970; by 2019, 67% of community hospitals were within systems.[20] Catholic hospitals top that with 96 to 98% of the acute, general Catholic hospitals being part of a system compared to 80% of non-Catholic similar hospitals (Table 5.1, Chapter 5).[12,22]

As hospitals formed systems, they also began to acquire other components of healthcare delivery, starting with physician practices, other care facilities, and insurance companies.[19] Initially, consolidations tended to be within a geographic region, but more recently, they have become cross-market, including across state lines.[20,21] This pattern played out with the large Catholic systems as well (see below). The preponderance of data demonstrates that these consolidations have increased costs and have had a mixed effect on quality of care.[19,21]

NON-FINANCIAL FORCES

As powerful as the financial forces have been in shaping healthcare, including Catholic healthcare, other non-financial forces were just as powerful (Table 7.1). The one that uniquely affected Catholic healthcare was the declining number of women religious. As presented in Chapters 2 and 3, it was these women who built (sometimes literally), ran, and funded the hospitals by doing everything from begging on the street to crafting innovative local insurance models. Their vows, including those of poverty and service, their sense of a calling to the poor, and their toughness imbued a special culture into Catholic healthcare.

In 1968, there were almost 180,000 women religious in numerous orders — an all-time high.[23] But this was not to continue. By 2021, that number had dropped to about 42,000, and their median age was 81 years old.[24] The enormous and abrupt loss of this group of unique, talented women leaders was caused by many women leaving the religious orders and many fewer entering. The reasons for this transformation reflect forces outside and inside the Church.[23]

This loss of women religious significantly changed the leadership of Catholic hospitals from the nuns to new lay administrators. While efforts were made by the various religious orders and the Catholic Health Association to inculcate the values and culture of the women religious into the new lay leaders, these leaders took no vows of obedience, poverty, or service; they may not have felt as deep a calling to the care of the poor; and probably had not been at the frontlines of care in their careers. How could this not have a profound effect on Catholic healthcare?

Other non-financial forces, including legislative and judicial actions and scientific advances, did not affect operations in the same way that leadership change did, but they brought into play the application and enforcement of the ERDs and their prohibitions, and shined a light on these prohibitions and their implications for patients (see Chapters 4 and 5).

The first of these legislative actions with an impact on Catholic healthcare was the legalization of contraception for married couples in 1965 and for all American women in 1972. Over the ensuing years, other actions with important implications for Catholic healthcare included the Supreme Court's *Roe v Wade* decision in 1973, affirming the Constitutional right of women to access abortion; its reversal with the *Dobbs* decision in 2022; medical-aid-in dying laws; and the series of actions that came under the rubric of "conscience objections" (see Chapter 6).

Scientific advances that enabled the prolongation of life and advances in reproductive technology were also factors that changed the healthcare landscape (see Chapter 5). Taken together, they set Catholic healthcare institutions apart from other healthcare institutions with regard to the care they could and would provide to Catholic and non-Catholic patients.

These combined financial and non-financial forces facilitated turning Catholic healthcare in America from small community hospitals whose clear mission was to care for the poor and vulnerable and that were owned and operated by nuns who were paid little or nothing, into corporate giants composed of multi-hospital systems sprawling across many states, managed by lay CEOs earning millions of dollars.

BECOMING CORPORATE

The United States is home to a number of very large Catholic healthcare systems. A Modern Healthcare ranking of healthcare systems in December 2021 listed six Catholic healthcare systems among the 25 largest healthcare systems in the country by operating revenue: CommonSpirit (#3), Providence (#4), Ascension (#5), Trinity (#7), Bon Secours Mercy Health (#21), and SSM Health (#24) (Table 7.2).[25] In a corrected list issued in March 2022, Bon Secours Mercy Health fell to #22, and SSM dropped off the list, falling just below #25. Nonetheless, SSM remains a large and important Catholic healthcare system and is discussed along with the others in this and subsequent chapters.

At the time of the March 2022 Modern Healthcare ranking, Intermountain Healthcare ranked #21, but it had not yet merged with a Catholic healthcare system to become Intermountain Health. The journey of each of these entities, including Intermountain Health, sheds light on the evolving structure, reach, and mission of Catholic healthcare in America.

The foundations of the large Catholic healthcare corporations were the many hospitals built by the nuns in the 1800s and early 1900s (see Chapters 2 and 3). The road from these initial small community hospitals to the current giant corporations was perhaps inevitable for Catholic hospitals, embedded as they were in America's capitalist healthcare system.

TABLE 7.2. Profiles of the Large Catholic Healthcare Systems

System	Rank[1]	Catholic Hosp (N)[2]	Total Hosp(N)[3]	Providers[3]	Employees[3]	States[3]
CommonSpirit	3	88	140	25,000[4]	150,000	21
Providence	4	38/45**	51	34,000[5]	117,000	7*
Ascension	5	79	139	36,000[6]	139,000	19(DC)
Trinity	7	47	88	27,000[7]	123,000	26
Bon Secours MH	21	44	48	3000[8]	60,000	7
SSM	24	23	23	12,800[9]	40,000	4

Information is from each system's websites unless otherwise indicated.
1. Ranking Modern Healthcare Dec 21,2021; Number Catholic hospitals (AHA); Total hospitals, Providers, and States with hospitals from the systems' websites
2. Hospital Operational and Demographic Data: *FY 2020 AHA Annual Survey Database.* Chicago: American Hospital Association, www.ahadata.com
3. Information on each systems website
4. Physicians and advanced practice clinicians; not indicated if employed or affiliated
5. Physicians; not indicated if employed or affiliate
6. Affiliated providers; 8300 employed providers
7. Physicians and clinicians; 7500 employed physicians and clinicians
8. Providers; not indicated if affiliated or employed
9. Providers; not indicated if affiliated or employed
* Some Providence data was personal communication Providence
**38 is from AHA data; 45 is from information supplied by Providence.

In some ways, it was a more straightforward and more obvious path for Catholic hospitals than for many other hospitals. There was a natural grouping of hospitals that were owned and operated by one or several groups of women religious who shared spiritual roots and a fervent desire to maintain the culture and mission of their institutions. Putting them under one umbrella with a corporate headquarters could create more uniformity and the potential for savings and enhanced revenue. Also, as the number of women religious decreased, one nun heading the corporation or a small group of nuns controlling a corporate board could leverage their influence over a number of hospitals.

However, over time, this movement toward horizontal consolidation went far beyond the union of Catholic hospitals run by one religious order or orders with a common heritage, to unions of hospitals owned by multiple orders, and then to unions with non-Catholic systems.

The mergers/affiliations that occurred with non-Catholic hospitals are in many ways surprising and hard to understand from the perspective of mission and value maintenance. Moreover, Part Six of the most recent version of the ERDs focused on such relationships with non-Catholic entities, discouraging them, forbidding the Catholic entity from profiting from activities deemed intrinsically immoral that are performed in the non-Catholic entity, and prohibiting the formation of an overarching organization to avoid compliance with the ERDs (see Chapter 4).[26]

How profits can be apportioned in a merged entity to avoid a Catholic entity from receiving any profits related to prohibited acts would seem to require financial contortions beyond even a creative CFO's imagination. Although the bishops of the diocese of the organizations involved must approve the structure of the relationship and guarantee that the ERDs are followed, it is not transparent or readily apparent how this is accomplished (see Chapter 4).

Often, the wording of the relationships seems carefully chosen to imply independence of the Catholic and non-Catholic entities. In fact, it might seem they are independent and not bound by the ERDs, which is desirable for patient access to the full range of healthcare services and physician autonomy, but in reality, the obligations to adhere to the ERDs may be there.

The path to Catholic healthcare becoming corporate behemoths may be best understood by examining in varying depth the journeys of the large Catholic systems that have put their footprint across America (Figure 5.1). The journeys have much in common: the coming together of hospitals run by one order of nuns; the joining of hospitals from other orders; the formation of a corporate entity, most often as a Catholic legal entity; and finally, the merging with non-Catholic partners. Also, there is almost always the acquisition of other healthcare entities — physician groups, insurance plans, urgent care centers, free-standing emergency departments, clinics, and long-term care facilities.

To gain insights into the outcome of these journeys, I sent a standardized questionnaire to executives of each of the large systems, except for Intermountain Health, as it had recently formed. Only SSM and Providence responded to the questionnaire, even sending additional information. Despite multiple requests, no response was received from CommonSpirit, Ascension, Trinity, or Bon Secours Mercy Health.

Intermountain Health

Of all the mergers that have occurred in Catholic healthcare, this is perhaps one of the most surprising and most telling regarding the current goals of Catholic healthcare and the application (or perhaps, more accurately, the non-application) of ERDs. Therefore, it is worth an in-depth look at its evolution.

Intermountain Health does not identify itself as a Catholic healthcare institution, and in many ways, it exemplifies the challenges and questions raised by mergers between Catholic and non-Catholic healthcare entities. Intermountain Health is the result of the merger of SCL Health, a Catholic system with hospitals in Colorado and Montana, and Intermountain Healthcare, a system with Mormon roots, based in Utah with healthcare facilities largely in Utah, Nevada, and Idaho.[27]

From a Catholic healthcare perspective, this merger is the culmination of a story of Catholic healthcare covering more than 150 years. It is representative of the journey of all the created systems.

The Kansas part of this story began in 1863 with the founding of St. John's Hospital in Leavenworth, Kansas, by the Sisters of Charity of Leavenworth, an offspring of the order founded by Mother Seton (see Chapters 2 and 3). In the ensuing 160 years, the sisters' healthcare mission extended across Kansas and into Nebraska, Wyoming, Montana, and Colorado, with hospitals springing up across the rugged West.[28,29] Many of the hospitals did not survive, but those that did became the foundation for the Catholic component of Intermountain Health.

The first step toward the Sisters of Charity of Leavenworth's hospitals becoming a corporate entity came in 1972, when the Articles of Incorporation for the Sisters of Charity of Leavenworth/Health Services Corporation, SCL/HSC, were filed, and Sister Mary Dennis became its first president.[29] The articulated benefits prompting the formation of the corporation were:

- To bring the hospitals into a unified system.
- To secure the assets of the Sisters of Charity of Leavenworth to provide for the needs of the sisters.
- To provide financial advantages to the hospitals, especially in their ability to access capital.
- To create better access to services such as group purchasing and consultative advice.[29]

Initially, the sisters established themselves as the dominant influence in the new entity, presumably with the intention of maintaining an ongoing commitment to the mission. The corporate board was the elected leaders of the Sisters of Charity of Leavenworth, and the individual hospitals' boards were required to have 51% of the members from the Sisters of Charity of Leavenworth.[30]

In 1994, a combined lay person and women religious board was formed, acknowledging the shifting leadership from the nuns to lay leaders.[30] Similarly, individual boards were then asked to have members from the Sister of Charity of Leavenworth only when women religious were available.[30]

Another corporate structure for the health system was created in 2011 with the transfer of SCL/HSC to the Leaven ministries (ministry is a term often used to describe a Catholic healthcare entity), which was a public juridic person.[30] This type of entity (which is not actually a person) is detailed in the canon law of the Catholic Church and comes under the Church hierarchy, but it also has civil status.[31]

Within canon law, juridic persons must have a purpose that is in accordance with the mission of the Church. It is a way to preserve the Catholic identity of an enterprise and its obligations to function within Catholic beliefs.[31] It has been stated that this is also a way to permit such an entity to *"remain free of civil law influences that can threaten the Catholicity...."*[31]

The Colorado part of the story, and ultimately the dominant part, began with St. Joseph's Hospital (initially called St. Vincent's Hospital) in Denver, Colorado, in 1873.[32] The sisters opened another hospital, St. Mary's, in 1896, across the Continental divide in Grand Junction, creating a needed place for care given the challenge patients had crossing the mountains to Denver.[33]

These hospitals were a response to a community's needs, but the hospitals, acquisitions, and relationships in more recent years appear to be based less on need and more on a corporate goal to expand the footprint and market share. In 1997, Lutheran Medical Center, a community hospital in the suburbs of Denver, joined St. Joseph's, which, along with a 120-member physician group, eventually formed Exempla Healthcare.[34]

The formal incorporation of St. Mary's in Grand Junction, the building of Good Samaritan in the Denver suburbs, and the incorporation of Platte Valley Medical Center into Exempla expanded the footprint significantly, contributing to the fact that 38% of the hospital beds in Colorado are under the Catholic umbrella, with all the attendant implications.[22]

The formal acquisition of Exempla by SCL Health in 2012 created a network of five Colorado and three Montana hospitals.[35] Subsequently, the Exempla name was dropped.

The expansion of the system's footprint did not stop. Across the Colorado state line was Intermountain Healthcare, which had been started by the Church of Jesus Christ of Latter-Day Saints. In 1975, the LDS Church turned over the healthcare system to Intermountain Healthcare.[36] In 2021, Intermountain Healthcare merged with SCL Health, creating one of the largest hospital systems in the mountain West, with healthcare facilities in Utah, Idaho, Nevada, Colorado, Kansas, Montana, and Wyoming.[37]

This new entity demonstrates that the reach of healthcare corporations extends well beyond the hospital walls. In 2022, the newly formed entity, Intermountain Health, not only owned 33 hospitals but also 385 clinics, a medical group with 3,800 physicians and advance care providers, an imaging center, home care, an insurance plan, and an emergency air service transport — fingers in every healthcare pie.[37]

What happened to SCL Health's Catholic identity and mission in this megamerger? Does Intermountain have any Catholic identity? These are interesting and important questions that apply not only to SCL Health and Intermountain Health, but also to every system we will examine. While the questions are clear, the answers are not, for Intermountain Health or any of the other systems.

As of December 2022, SCL Health's landing page did not mention that it is Catholic. If one clicks on the "About Us" button, one learns that it is faith-based. One can then click on the Catholic healthcare link to find out that they follow the ERDs, and one can click again to a link to the United States Council of Catholic Bishops to learn about the ERDs.

As of June 2023, there is a new website that only has Intermountain Healthcare on the landing page — SCL is not mentioned except at the very bottom as "an equal opportunity employer."[38] Exploring the "About Us" section supplies the same information as previously.[38]

The Archbishop of Denver, who has responsibility for the maintenance of SCL Catholic beliefs, asserts its commitment to the ERDs (see below). However, it is unclear if the ERDS are enforced for SCL members who are not Catholic. If one goes to the website of Platte Valley Medical Center, which is a member of SCL Health, one finds that its landing page describes the medical center as a secular member affiliated with SCL Health.[39] Not surprisingly, Intermountain Health's landing page has no mention of Catholic healthcare.

Some services that are not permitted by the ERDs, including contraception, IVF, and gender-affirming care, are available at Intermountain facilities, and these services generate revenue for the system.[37] This raises the question of how the revenues from these services are walled off from the Catholic components as required by the ERDs.

Intermountain Health will not be discussed further as the entity is too recently formed to have information that is comparable to that of the other systems.

CommonSpirit Health

CommonSpirit Health was formed in 2019 as the final step in a series of consolidations of hospitals and health systems established by Catholic women religious congregations across the nation. CommonSpirit Health describes itself as *"the alignment of Catholic Health Initiatives (CHI) and Dignity Health."*[40] Alignment is one of those terms used for these new Catholic healthcare corporations that leaves one wondering about the actual relationship between the entities and whether they are a Catholic system or not.

CHI was formed in 1996 by the merger of the Franciscan Health System and Sisters of Charity Health Care System that were fruits of 13 religious congregations. Other Catholic healthcare systems and religious communities later joined, and eventually, non-Catholic systems were woven into the corporation of 100 hospitals in 17 states.[41]

CHI was a public juridic person with both lay and religious leadership. CHI's headquarters were in Colorado, where it operated the Centura system that had hospitals across Colorado, a number of which had been established by religious congregations in the late 1800s. In 1996, when Centura became part of CHI, it also created a union with the Adventist healthcare system (a non-Catholic Church religiously operated system), which operated five hospitals in Colorado, bringing the system to 13 Colorado hospitals.[42]

This union suddenly dissolved without any explanation in 2023, with the Adventist system no longer being part of CommonSpirit Health.[43] However, Centura/CHI apparently had no intention of becoming a smaller organization or not compete with Intermountain Health's Colorado-Utah links. One day after the split with the Adventist system, Centura/CHI announced the acquisition of five hospitals in Utah, extending its geographic footprint in the West and placing Catholic hospitals in that state where none had been previously.[44]

Dignity's story has an interesting twist. Dignity's foundation stone was St. Mary's Hospital in San Francisco, which was founded by the Sisters of Mercy and opened in 1857. The initial incarnation of Dignity was as Catholic Healthcare West, which was the result of the two separate congregations of the Sisters of Mercy joining together their 10 hospitals.[45]

In 2012, Catholic Health West changed not only its name, but also its core Catholic identity, becoming Dignity Health. It was no longer an official ministry of the Catholic Church and became an institution *"rooted in Catholic tradition."* Dignity's website claims, *"We changed our name to Dignity Health to better describe what we stand for."*[45] However, it is not clear what that means. It seems more likely that this change was done to free the 15 non-Catholic hospitals from at least some of the care limitations of the ERDs, while maintaining others (see Chapter 5). Dignity's hospitals operate under what has been dubbed "A Statement of Common Values." It states,

> *"For Dignity Health, respecting the dignity of persons requires reverence at every stage of life's journey from conception to natural death. Therefore, direct abortion is not performed. Reproductive technologies in which conception occurs outside a woman's body will not be part of Dignity Health's services. This includes in-vitro fertilization... Death is a sacred part of life's journey; we will intentionally neither hasten nor delay it. For this reason, physician-assisted suicide is not part of Dignity Health's mission."*[45]

By omission, this seems to permit some other services prohibited under the ERDs and other Catholic prohibitions, such as contraception and gender-affirming care.

CommonSpirit emerged as a complicated amalgam. CommonSpirit Health is composed of 138 hospitals (other parts of the website state 139 or 140) and more than 1,000 care sites in urban and rural areas in 21 states, not all of which have a hospital facility, including Washington, Oregon, California, Nevada, Arizona, New Mexico, Colorado, Texas, Arkansas, Kansas, Nebraska, Iowa, Minnesota, North Dakota, Wisconsin, Indiana, Ohio, Tennessee, Georgia, Kentucky, and West Virginia. (There is some difference in the states pictured on the landing page and the sites of employment).[40]

This extensive network has 150,000 employees and 25,000 physicians and advance practice clinicians. CommonSpirit's Organized Health Care Arrangements include senior living facilities, skilled nursing facilities, home care, and hospices.[40] CommonSpirit states that it provides care for 20 million patients and that one in every four Americans has access to care in one of its facilities.[40]

This enormous reach geographically and in the points and types of care underscores the importance of policymakers and the public understanding the limitations of care in a Catholic system and in the transparency regarding it.

Although CommonSpirit is the corporate entity, as of July 2023, the hospitals in the system maintain the logos and names of the original component systems. For example, on the website landing page for St. Mary's in San Francisco, the name and logo reference Dignity, and there is no mention of CommonSpirit.[46] Similarly, CHI Health Creighton University Medical Center in Nebraska displays on its landing page the CHI name and logo.[47] The Colorado hospital members display the Centura logo and name.[48] Virginia Mason Medical Center displays its Franciscan identity.[49] This seems less than transparent about ownership, relationships, and identity.

Although CommonSpirit Health is described as a Catholic healthcare system, reflecting the ambiguity noted above, neither the website landing page nor the "Mission, Values, and Vision" link states that it or any component of the system is Catholic.[40] However, the "Working Here" section, which lists job openings across the enterprise, indicates it is a Catholic system; this includes job openings in states that are in the Dignity component of the system.[40] While no part of the main website indicates that the system abides by ERDs or links to them, the "Working Here" section states that employees must follow the ERDs.[40]

During the planning phase of the CHI and Dignity merger, even the bioethicists appear to have been confused about the entity's religious identity. There was a question of whether CommonSpirit Health "was Catholic enough" to obtain the necessary Vatican approval. The president of the National Catholic Bioethics Center rendered an unfavorable moral approval. Subsequently, CHI and Dignity sought additional moral analyses from three other ethicists, who gave favorable opinions.[50]

The ERDs require that the bishops overseeing the dioceses in which the institutions reside guarantee compliance with the ERDs (see Chapter 4). Archbishops of Denver and San Francisco would have been those bishops, and they approved the merger. The Vatican agreed that it was their decision.

In response to a letter I wrote to the Archbishop of Denver regarding this merger and the SCL Intermountain Health merger, his office confirmed "*...that we were involved in the discussions surrounding the merger of CHI with Dignity Health and the recent merger of SCL Health with Intermountain. Without breaking confidentiality, I can say that Archbishop Aquila has been adamant in conversations with the leadership of these systems that the ERDs be followed.*" (Personal communication, David Uebbing, Archbishop Aquila's office, January 23, 2023.)

However, it appears that even those with close working relationships with the Dignity component of CommonSpirit do not know if it is Catholic and whether or not they are following the ERDs. This is reflected by the efforts of the physician faculty of the University of California Health System wanting clarification in contracts with Dignity and other Catholic providers that the physicians will be able to use their judgment in patient care and not be constrained by ERDs.[51]

If ethicists and physicians are unsure and if the websites are confusing, how can patients ascertain if their care is at a Catholic institution that abides by the ERDs or at one that does not adhere to care prohibitions? The simple answer appears to be that they cannot.

Providence St. Joseph Health Care

Providence (Providence St. Joseph), one of the largest Catholic healthcare systems, grew from the early efforts of Mother Joseph and the Sisters of Providence (see Chapters 2 and 3) in the Northwest and the later efforts of the Sisters of St. Joseph of Orange in California.

Mother Joseph opened the first hospital in the Northwest in 1858: St. Joseph's Hospital in Vancouver, Washington (see Chapters 2 and 3).[52] The evolution of the system is well-detailed on the websites of Providence Health Care and the Providence Archives. Much of the information detailed here comes from those sources.[53,54]

In the late 1800s, 12 additional hospitals were established in Washington, Montana, and Oregon[54]; six hospitals were established in Washington, Oregon, Alaska, and California in the first half of the 1900s.[54] The second half of the 1900s was marked by relinquishing some of the hospitals to other entities and assuming management or sponsorship of other Catholic and non-Catholic hospitals, and the establishment of a health plan.

In 2006, Providence Health & Services was formed, providing healthcare in Washington, Montana, Oregon, Alaska, and California.[54] In 2010,

Providence Ministries became a public juridic person sponsoring Providence Health & Services.[54] In 2012, Providence affiliated with Swedish Health Services, a major non-Catholic health care system in Seattle.[54] In 2014, Providence affiliated with a large, multispecialty medical group, Pacific Medical Center, agreeing that the Pacific Medical Center physicians did not need to follow the ERDs.[55]

How these arrangements conform to the ERD requirements and were approved by the bishop is not clear. It is of note that Providence lists Swedish Health Service in Seattle and Covent Health in Texas and New Mexico as "affiliate family"—another ambiguous designation.[53]

The Sisters of St. Joseph of Orange is one of the many congregations of the Sisters of St. Joseph in the United States. Following their work in the 1918 flu epidemic in California in 1920, they opened St. Joseph's Hospital in Eureka, California, and in 1929, added St. Joseph's Hospital in Orange, California. In 2016, Providence Health & Services merged with St. Joseph's Health, forming Providence St. Joseph's Health.[53]

Providence operates 51 acute general hospitals in Washington, Alaska, Montana, Oregon, and California. Through their "affiliate family," they reach into Texas and New Mexico. Forty-five of the system's hospitals are Catholic and adhere to the ERDs; the secular healthcare facilities do not follow the ERDs. The system includes five free-standing emergency departments, 81 urgent care facilities, 24 assisted living facilities, 16 supportive housing ministries, and a health plan. The system employs 117,000 individuals and has 34,000 physicians. The physicians are permitted to refer patients for procedures not offered in a given facility. (Information in this paragraph is from the Providence website and personal communication, Adrienne Webb, Providence.)[53]

Providence's main landing page and the "About Us" link do not list its Catholic identity or that it abides by the ERDs, nor is there a link to the ERDs.[53] Its annual report to the community does not indicate that it is Catholic.[53] Examination of the website landing pages of four Providence hospitals on January 18, 2023, showed that none of them indicated that they are Catholic institutions.

Ascension Health

Ascension was formed by a series of hospital mergers and acquisitions starting in 1999 with the joining of the Daughters of Charity National Health System and the Sisters of St. Joseph Health System.[56] Later, the health systems of other religious communities and non-Catholic systems became part of Ascension. There were five sponsoring religious orders, including a men's religious order, the Congregation of Alexian Brothers.

The Alexian Brothers is one of the few male religious orders that contributed to the growth of healthcare in America. Their story began in Europe in 1259, with their care of the sick and burial of the dead.[57] Members of their order arrived in the United States in 1866 and started a hospital in Chicago for boys and men. They subsequently started other hospitals in Missouri, Wisconsin, and New Jersey.[57]

Ascension Health is a ministerial public juridic person. The system includes 139 hospitals in 19 states and the District of Columbia; 2,600 sites of care, including 39 senior living facilities in 11 states and the District of Columbia; a home health service; an insurance plan; and a billion-dollar venture capital fund.[56] The system has 139,000 employees and 8,300 employed providers.[56]

Ascension's landing page affirms its Catholic identity. The "Mission, Vision, Values and Equity" section also notes its Catholic identity. It states that its *"Healthcare ethics focuses on supporting personalized care that is consistent with each patient's individual values and promotes the good of the human person."*[56] One could argue that this is a misstatement given that as a Catholic system, the care is guided by the ERDs and not the patient's values or shared decision-making.

The websites of at least some of its hospitals have a common design but provide less information on the specific hospital than the primary Ascension site. None that were examined noted that they were Catholic. To find that out, one has to go to the bottom of the page, which is devoted to the Ascension system, and click on "About Us."

Trinity Health

Trinity Health was formed in 2013 by the merger of Trinity Health and Catholic Health East.[58] These two systems were the product of previous mergers of hospitals and health systems built by four orders of women religious: the Congregation of the Sisters of Holy Cross, the Sisters of Mercy of the Americas, the Franciscan Sisters of Allegany, and the Sisters of Providence of Holyoke. Information on Trinity Health and the founding religious communities is available on the respective websites.[58,59]

The Sisters of the Holy Cross arrived in America in Indiana in 1843.[59] Their entrance into healthcare began in 1861 with the care of soldiers during the Civil War. This experience led them to provide nursing care in hospitals in Kentucky, Illinois, Tennessee, Missouri, and Washington, DC. The Sisters established 19 hospitals.[59] In 1979, they consolidated their healthcare organizations into the Holy Cross Health System.

Sisters of Mercy of the Americas, who also came to America in 1843, opened their first hospital in Pittsburgh, Pennsylvania, in 1847 (see Chapter 2). The multiple chapters of the order established hospitals in Maryland, New York, Maine, Georgia, Florida, Iowa, and California.

Trinity's legal sponsor is Catholic Health Ministries, a public juridic person. The system operates in 26 states with 88 hospitals, 136 urgent care facilities, 135 care facilities, senior care facilities that include living facilities and skilled nursing, home care, and a specialty pharmacy.[58] Trinity employs 123,000 individuals and 7,500 employed physicians and clinicians and has affiliation with 27,000 physicians and clinicians.[58] Trinity's leadership intends to follow the overall industry and shift inpatient care to ambulatory care and to expand home health, urgent care, specialty pharmacy, and telehealth.[60]

Although Trinity Health's landing page does not say it is Catholic, the "About Us" section indicates that it is. However, neither that section nor the section on "Mission, Values and Vision" indicates that Trinity complies with the ERDs, nor does it link to them.[58]

Examination of the websites on January 18, 2023, of eight Trinity Hospitals in six states did not reveal any consistency in stating their Catholic identity. None stated on the landing page they were Catholic; three noted the religious orders that founded the hospitals; and two had a link to the main Trinity website.

Holy Cross Hospital's website landing page does not indicate if it is Catholic or if it follows the ERDs. This is relevant given its emphasis on maternity care, stating it *"delivers more babies and cares for more newborns with complex medical issues than any other hospital in Maryland or the District of Columbia, and is among the largest single-site hospital providers of obstetric services in the United States."*[61]

Trinity Health Ann Arbor, Michigan, which is one of the largest Trinity hospitals, does not mention that it is Catholic, nor does the link provided to Trinity for "Mission and Values" and "Vision."

Bon Secours Mercy Health

Bon Secours Mercy Health was established in 2018 by the merger of Bon Secours Health System and Mercy Health.[63] These two systems were built by three women religious orders: the Sisters of Bon Secours, the Sisters of Mercy, and the Sisters of the Humility of Mary.[63] The details of the health system and the religious orders are provided on their respective websites and the archives of the religious orders, from which many of the following details are taken.

Although the Sisters of Bon Secours started their ministry with home care (see Chapter 2), they did not abandon the use of hospitals. In 1919, the sisters opened their first hospital in Baltimore and others followed in Washington, DC, Michigan, Massachusetts, and Virginia. In 1983, their healthcare operations were unified as Bon Secours Health System.[64]

Mercy Health was formed by the coming together of several religious orders. It was initially established in 1986 by the health ministries of the regional communities of the Sisters of Mercy.[65] The orders' first hospitals were opened in Ohio and Pennsylvania in the mid to late 1800s. Subsequently, the Sisters of Humility of Mary and the Franciscan Sisters of the Poor joined their healthcare efforts with those of the Sisters of Mercy. Following the union of the hospitals of the religious orders, non-Catholic hospitals were incorporated into the system.

Bon Secours Mercy Health includes facilities in Florida, Kentucky, Maryland, New York, Ohio, South Carolina, and Virginia, including 48 hospitals, free-standing emergency departments, imaging centers, and healthcare-related businesses, including a private equity portfolio and a digital innovation group.[63] The system employs 60,000 people and has 3,000 providers.[63]

Although the Bon Secours Mercy Health website landing page states that it has a Catholic heritage, it does not state that it is a Catholic healthcare institution, nor does it indicate if it adheres to the ERDs or provide a link to them.

SSM Health

SSM is the smallest of the major Catholic healthcare systems and, in some ways, the "most Catholic." The story of its evolution is detailed on its website, and much of the historical information below is from that site.[66]

Unlike the other major Catholic healthcare systems, SSM has woven together only Catholic healthcare institutions. These were started by four separate groups of nuns: the Franciscan Sisters of Mary; their offshoot, the Sisters of St. Francis; the Sisters of St. Agnes; and the Felician Sisters.[66]

The Franciscan Sisters of Mary and their founder, Mother Mary Odilia Berger, are detailed in Chapters 2 and 3. In 1877, they founded St. Mary's Infirmary in St. Louis, which became the cornerstone for SSM (see Chapter 2). A group of Sisters left the St. Louis congregation in 1894 to strike out on their own. Five years later, they started the first hospital in the Oklahoma territory, St. Anthony's Hospital, followed by hospitals in Wisconsin. St. Anthony's remains an important component of SSM and is its largest hospital.[66]

The Sisters of St. Agnes began providing healthcare in 1896, opening hospitals and clinics in Wisconsin and Illinois. Their system became Agnesian Healthcare. The Felician Sisters' healthcare work spanned 10 states and parts of Canada.[66]

SSM Health emerged in 1986–1987, bringing all the healthcare operations of the reunited Franciscan Sisters of St. Mary and Sisters of St. Francis (now the Franciscan Sisters of Mary). Sister Mary Jean Ryan was the first CEO. The system grew with the incorporation of Agnesian HealthCare and the development of a joint operating agreement with the Felician Sisters for some of their hospitals.[66]

As with other Catholic healthcare systems, the role of the women religious decreased with time. In 2011, the first lay CEO was appointed. In 2013, the sponsorship of SSM was transferred from the Franciscan Sisters of Mary to SSM Health Ministries, a public juris person with both lay persons and religious women overseeing its operation.[66]

SSM Health's landing page does not indicate that it is Catholic, but the "Mission, Values, and Vision" states that it is a Catholic entity and is the only one of the major Catholic healthcare systems that states that "*As a Catholic organization, SSM Health operates in alignment with the Ethical and Religious Directives for Catholic Health Care Services.*"[66] Moreover, it provides a direct link to the Sixth Edition of the ERDs — the only major Catholic system with this level of transparency. An examination of the websites of four SSM hospitals in four states, however, showed that none indicated they were Catholic institutions, but the SSM system link to "Mission, Values, and Vision" is provided and is as described above.

As of 2022, SSM operates 23 hospitals in Missouri, Wisconsin, Oklahoma, and Illinois. SSM also operates a health plan, 149 urgent care centers, six free-standing emergency departments, seven senior living facilities, 13 post-acute facilities, home health services, a pharmacy benefit corporation, and an insurance plan. SSM employs 40,000 individuals and has 12,800 providers.

All the hospitals, urgent care centers, and emergency departments comply with the ERDs. The physicians cannot refer to providers for treatments prohibited under the ERDs (Information in this paragraph is from SSM website and personal communication Patrick Kampert, SSM).[66]

A BUMP IN THE FINANCIAL ROAD

Most hospitals and healthcare systems, including the large Catholic systems, that had been amassing profits over a number of successive years hit a rough patch recently. In fiscal year 2022, CommonSpirit experienced a $1.85 billion operating loss compared to a $5.45 billion net gain in the previous year.[67]

Providence ended its 2022 fiscal year with a $1.7 billion operating loss and a $6.1 billion net loss, compared to a net income of $812 million in 2021.[68] Ascension closed its 2022 fiscal year with an operating loss of $879 million, a net loss of more than $1.8 billion, compared to an almost $5.7 billion net gain the previous year.[69] Trinity Health had a net loss of $1.4 billion for its fiscal year that ended June 33, 2022.[70] This followed a previous particularly good year with nearly $3.9 billion in net income.[70]

Bon Secours Mercy Health posted a $1.2 billion net loss in 2022, compared to a $997.7 million gain the year before.[71] SSM lost $484 million in nine months that ended September 2022, compared to a gain of $447.5 million in the same period the year before.[72]

These losses reflected an increase in labor and supply costs, decreased government relief payments, and large investment losses.[67-70] However, 2023 appears to be putting them back on track for profits. Although hospitals, in general, experienced better financial performance in January 2023 than in the previous January, none of them see 2023 as a return to the "golden years" quite yet.[73]

CONCLUSION

American healthcare has been radically transformed over the decades from doctor's offices and small community hospitals into today's medical-industrial complex of large healthcare systems. These systems have employed and affiliated physicians and a range of vertically integrated services with free-standing emergency departments, urgent care centers, imaging and ambulatory surgery centers, emergency transport services, insurance plans, senior living facilities, pharmacy benefit organizations, and even venture capital companies.

Healthcare has moved from a truly nonprofit enterprise, often relying on philanthropy, to highly profitable, rich enterprises. Catholic hospitals have not been immune from this transformation. They are now some of the largest, wealthiest healthcare systems in the United States.

The journeys of the seven large systems paint a complex and, at times, confusing picture of the transformation of Catholic healthcare in America. The nuns who built the hospitals are gone, replaced by lay administrators. Catholic hospitals merged with non-Catholic hospitals, making it virtually impossible to know if your hospital is Catholic or not and what that means.

These new entities are sprawling corporations that reach across states and state lines and across the entire healthcare terrain. They have placed their stamp on all American healthcare. Millions of Americans, Catholic and non-Catholic, from the heartlands to the coasts, rely on them for their care. Policymakers need to understand the implications of this reach. Catholics need to ask, "Has the mission at the heart of Catholic healthcare been maintained, or has it been lost, replaced by more corporate goals?"

CHAPTER 8

Mission Fidelity

For where your treasure is there will your heart be also.
                                                Jesus, Matthew 6:21

The mission for Catholic healthcare is a complex blend of remaining true to its biblical roots, obeying the Church's rules, and fulfilling its societal and legal obligations — not an easy path. Although each of these components places somewhat different burdens on Catholic healthcare, they all intersect at the care of the poor and most vulnerable.

Judaic-Christian teaching has a deep theological and historical commitment to healing of those in need — even those who are not in our own religious tent (Chapter 1). For Catholicism, Jesus' healing ministry, given freely to all, especially to the poor and those marginalized by society, became the template for Catholic healthcare for almost two millennia. The beginning of Catholic healthcare in America was most notable for its laser focus on care for the most vulnerable, the immigrants, and the poor (Chapter 2). The care was given selflessly by women religious whose personal payment was spiritual, not material (Chapters 2 and 3). They did not desire or attempt to build large fortunes for the institutions.

Not only must Catholic healthcare uphold this past, but currently, it must abide by the many components of the ERDs, the first of which is care for the poor (Chapter 4). As healthcare institutions, they have an obligation to provide high-quality care to those who walk through their doors. As not-for-profit healthcare institutions, they must fulfill a commitment to support their community in return for their tax benefits. To assess if Catholic healthcare has mission fidelity, each of these dimensions must be examined.

MISSION STATEMENTS

Mission statements are thoughtfully crafted and reflect an organization's core identity commitments. Therefore, it is useful to review the mission statements of the major Catholic healthcare systems as an initial step in assessing mission fidelity. As we would expect, the mission statements center on God, Jesus, and the Gospel, and focus on the poor and the vulnerable.

Ascension: "*Rooted in the loving ministry of Jesus as healer, we commit ourselves to serving all persons with special attention to those who are poor and vulnerable. Our Catholic health ministry is dedicated to spiritually centered, holistic care which sustains and improves the health of individuals and communities. We are advocates for a compassionate and just society through our actions and our words.*"[1]

Bon Secours Mercy Health: "*Our mission is to extend the compassionate ministry of Jesus by improving the health and well-being of our communities and bring good help to those in need, especially people who are poor, dying and underserved.*"[2]

CommonSpirit Health: "*As CommonSpirit Health, we make the healing presence of God known in our world by improving the health of the people we serve, especially those who are vulnerable, while we advance social justice for all.*"[3]

Providence: "*As expressions of God's healing love, witnessed through the ministry of Jesus, we are steadfast in serving all, especially those who are poor and vulnerable.*"[4]

SSM Health: "*Through our exceptional health care services, we reveal the healing presence of God.*"[5]

Trinity Health: "*We, Trinity Health, serve together in the spirit of the Gospel as a compassionate and transforming healing presence within our communities.*"[6]

CARE FOR THE POOR AND VULNERABLE

These mission statements are admirable and uplifting, but are they being operationalized? Do they truthfully represent what these healthcare systems do?

A good starting place to assess the validity of the mission statements is with how these systems treat the patients who cannot afford care in their institutions. In 2021, 27.5 million non-elderly adults were uninsured in America.[7] An additional 34% of working-age adults either did not have insurance for the entire year or were inadequately insured in 2022.[8] These patients still get sick and need care. Sixty-one percent of underinsured individuals simply avoid needed care — an unfortunate choice.[8]

However, when uninsured and underinsured patients do opt to obtain care, they often find themselves in debt. Half the individuals in a Commonwealth survey said they would be unable to pay for an unexpected medical bill of $1,000 within 30 days.[8] Overall, 10% of Americans have medical debt; 30% of the underinsured or intermittently uninsured had been turned over to a collection agency; and 58% of all debt collection is medical debt.[8,9] Not surprisingly, 21% of people in poor health and 15% of people with disability have medical debt.[9]

So, what do hospitals do and, more importantly, what should they do for these patients who need care, but who can't afford it and/or find themselves owing money when they do get needed healthcare?

In keeping with the general approach in healthcare, hospitals can and should put in place preventive measures that help patients obtain affordable care and avoid garnering debt. They can help eligible patients enroll in insurance coverage such as Medicaid. They can provide robust financial aid programs that are easily and transparently available. They can have a sliding fee scale based on patients' ability to pay.

But what if prevention was never instituted or failed? What happens when patients accrue unpaid medical bills? In the latter situation, some hospitals develop a reasonable repayment plan, but the repayment can stretch for years.

Given the pervasiveness and impact of medical debt, KFF News undertook an extensive investigation of hospitals' debt collection policies and practices by reviewing written policies, making telephone calls, sending emails, and conducting interviews to get a picture of what hospitals say or don't say and what they do or don't do.[10] The researchers focused on four specific policies:

- Reporting to credit agencies.
- Selling patient debt.
- Taking a range of legal actions.
- Denying non-emergency care.

What they found among hospitals for which policies were available is concerning[10]:

- More than two-thirds report patients to credit agencies.
- A quarter sell the patients' debts to debt collectors.
- More than two-thirds sue patients or pursue actions such as garnishing their wages or placing liens on their property.

- About 20% deny non-emergency care to patients if they owe the hospital payments.
- Almost 40% are not transparent about what they do.
- There is often a disconnect between hospital policies and what spokespeople say are actual practices.

All these actions can and do wreak havoc in the patients' lives, often for years.

One would hope that Catholic hospitals aggressively pursue every preventive measure and have policies that do not permit these actions. News reports and detailed studies suggest that this hope may not be realized.

The KFF News examined the policies in 528 hospitals, some of which were Catholic.[10] Of course, the presence of a policy does not mean policies are implemented in all or any instances.

The hospitals in the Ascension and Trinity systems had the most aggressive reported policies. Ascension's policies permitted all four actions; however, a spokesperson for Ascension said none of these are current practice.[10]

The policies in the Trinity hospital system permitted three of the four practices,[10] but Trinity officials did not respond to repeated questions from KFF News about whether hospitals in the systems sell patient debt.[10] It seems especially far afield from their missions if Catholic hospitals' policies permit the denial of non-emergency care to patients.

The CHI and the Dignity hospitals under the CommonSpirit umbrella reported policies that allowed credit reporting and selling of debt but did not permit denial of non-emergency care or legal action.[10] However, as with Ascension, the system's spokesperson stated the credit reporting and debt collection were not current practice. Nonetheless their preventive measures in some instances seem wanting, at least in the past.

In 2017, the state of Washington sued CHI Franciscan, a part of CommonSpirit, for not offering charity care as required; the system provided patients with $22 million in debt relief and refunds because of the state action.[11]

The single Providence hospital in the KFF News study allowed none of the practices, but the Providence system was also sued by the state of Washington and was the focus of a *New York Times* report on aggressive debt collection (see below).[10,12]

In 2022, the *New York Times* did a series of articles on "Profit Over Patients." One might have expected that the spotlight would have been on for-profit hospitals, but no. Each of the articles detailed different concerning behaviors by a Catholic healthcare system. These included utilizing special drug pricing available to a hospital in a poor neighborhood to benefit a highly profitable system, aggressive billing practices, and major staff reductions to grow the bottom line.[12-14] None of these practices are unique to these systems.

The coverage of Bon Secours Mercy Health painted a picture of "taking from the poor to give to the rich."[13] The following details are from the *New York Times*' article. Bon Secours Mercy Health has the highest profit margins of all the Virginia hospitals, generating $100 million in a year.[13] The investigation attests that Bon Secours Mercy Health used the federal program intended for purchasing drugs for the poor (340B program) to fill its pharmacies with drugs that it could then dispense at a higher price to the insurers of patients who were not in need, generating system income.[13]

The use of this program was enabled by buying Richmond Community Hospital in 1995—a hospital in a poor part of town that was facing financial stress.[13] Bon Secours Mercy Health stated they had provided nearly $10 million in improvements to the hospital and invested nearly $9 million in the community.[13] This would have been a wonderful story had it continued. However, it seems those investments did not continue. Also, parts of the hospital, including the small five-bed ICU, were closed, turning the facility into what community members saw as more of an urgent care facility than a hospital.[13]

Of course, closing a small ICU may have been justified on the basis of patient volume, availability of staffing, or quality. Moreover, Bon Secours Mercy Health is certainly not the only hospital system that has used the 340B program outside its intended use.[15] But as a large Catholic system, should the bar be higher for Bon Secours Mercy Health? It is a question of mission fidelity. Do these actions reflect the statement made in the *Baltimore Sun* when the Sisters of Bon Secours first came to America they are *"waiting the call of those who may need their experience and services, without money and without price"*?[16]

Another piece in the *New York Times* series of focused the spotlight on Providence's aggressive billing practices.[12] The details here are from that article.

One of the practices reported was the intent and content of the training that the hospital staff received to obtain payments from patients. In part in response to rising costs of "free care," Providence paid McKinsey $45 million to help with a program called "Rev-Up" which included a training session entitled "Don't Accept the First No."[12] The training material explains that the patients should be told they may be eligible for financial assistance only as a last resort.[12] A spokesperson for Providence stated that the intent of Rev-Up was "*not to target or pressure those in financial distress. We recognize the tone of the training materials …was not consistent with our values.*"[12] She stated the materials have been modified to ensure compassion and respect in their communication.

It is important to underscore that in Washington state, where Providence is headquartered, hospitals are required to provide free care for anyone whose income is below 300% of the federal poverty level, which is $83,250 for a family of four.[12] The Attorney General of the state believed Providence violated this law, claiming that debt collectors were used for 55,000 patients who Providence stated owed them $73 million.[12] At that time, Providence had revenue in excess of $27 billion.[12] This led a former Providence employee to state, "*It was awful working for this rich system and not being able to help people who were just crying in front of me.*"[12]

Again, Providence is not the only hospital that takes this kind of action; however, is there a higher bar for them? Is this mission fidelity? How does this comport with the spirit of Providence's founder, Mother Joseph, who went on "begging tours" across the wilds of the West to pay for patient care? (see Chapter 3). Providence leadership may have decided it does not, since a spokesperson for Providence said, "*Providence has also instructed the debt collection firms it works with to not use 'any aggressive tactics such as garnishing wages or reporting delinquent accounts to credit agencies.'*"[12]

The third Catholic healthcare system profiled by the *New York Times* series of "Profit Over Patients" was Ascension for its cost-cutting in pursuit of higher revenue that may have contributed to a shortage of nurses in at least some of its hospitals.[14] The details below are from that article.

In 2013, concerned about impending losses, Ascension laid off about 3% of its staff, including nurses.[14] Ascension's leaders stated that their "Successful Labor Optimization Efforts" produced almost $500 million in savings over three years.[14] However, this may have resulted in some undesirable consequences: shortages of nurses, unfilled shifts, too few nurses at the bedside, and nurses being asked to work 16-hour shifts.[14]

These issues may have been part of the reason for the recent lawsuit filed by four Illinois nurses against Ascension as well as the nurses' strike at a number of Ascension hospitals in June 2023.[17,18]

While cutting costs, Ascension amassed $18 billion in cash reserves and has an investment company that managed over $41 billion.[14] Once again, Ascension is not alone in this behavior of cutting staff to shore up the bottom line, but the same question arises for them as for Bon Secours Mercy Health and Providence of mission fidelity: "How does this fit with the credos of their founders and their own mission statement?"

Another yardstick to assess a healthcare organization's commitment to care for the poor and vulnerable is the percentage of patients it cares for whose insurance coverage is Medicaid, as this is the government program designed for patients in poverty and/or vulnerable — patients specifically mentioned in the mission statement of four of the six systems. Medicaid's payments are lower than commercial insurance payments, so these are not patients whom hospitals seek out or even welcome. The Community Catalyst found that the Catholic hospitals had a lower percentage of discharged patients with Medicaid insurance coverage than other not-for-profit or for-profit acute general hospitals: 7.2 %, 8.3% and 9.0% of discharges, respectively.[19]

Patients with no insurance are rarely welcomed by any hospital except safety net hospitals. Ninety-nine of 417 non-critical access Catholic hospitals indicated they had a specific indigent care clinic.[20] The intent of this 24% of Catholic hospitals with the clinics could be interpreted in two ways: (1) that the hospital is indeed making a specific commitment to these patients, reflecting mission fidelity for this small group of hospitals; or (2) that the hospitals with the clinics wished to segregate these patients from others and limit available appointments.

Another service that can indicate a commitment to uninsured patients is an enrollment assistance program that facilitates patients gaining access to insurance coverage, including the hospital's financial assistance program — a debt prevention measure. Two hundred seventy-eight of 417 non-critical access Catholic hospitals (67%) indicated they had such a program.[20] However, having programs for financial assistance does not mean they will be earnestly brought to the patients' attention.

All hospitals are part of a community, and they should be especially committed to serving it. Given their history and responsibilities under the ERDs, Catholic hospitals and healthcare systems should be particularly attuned to serving the most vulnerable in their neighborhood. This can be measured by examining the characteristics of the patient population served by the hospital with regard to race, income, and education, in comparison to those characteristics of the population in a hospital's service area. The Lown Institute Hospital Index has measured this as an indication of community inclusivity for hospitals and systems (Table 8.1).[21] Among the large systems, SSM was the only one ranking in the top 100 systems (top tertile) for inclusivity, ranking number 29.

TABLE 8.1. Lown Institute Hospital Index Rankings for Catholic Healthcare Systems

Category	Ascension	Bon Secours MH	CommonSpirit	Providence	SSM	Trinity
Overall	170	106	68	96	90	67
Patient Outcome	162	90	69	28	205	89
Patient Safety	99	191	112	69	212	172
Avoiding Overuse	203	221	179	100	142	106
Inclusivity	113	119	151	254	29	178
Community Benefit	134	165	161	158	180	140

Data source: Lown Institute Hospital Index. https://lowninstitute.org/projects/lown-institute-hospitals-index
Accessed July 2023
296 systems were ranked.

COMMUNITY BENEFIT

The overwhelming majority of Catholic hospitals are not-for-profit institutions. As such, they receive substantial tax exemptions from federal income tax, state corporate income tax, state and local sales tax, and local property tax. They also can finance construction and other capital projects with lower rates using tax-exempt bonds. The tax benefit to not-for-profit hospitals is considerable, calculated to be nearly $28 billion in 2020; $14.5 billion is the value of the federal tax exemption and $13.2 billion is the value of state and local tax exemptions.[22]

In return for this government support, not-for-profit hospitals, including the Catholic hospitals, are required to give back to the communities in which they reside. They can accomplish this requirement in a variety of ways.

A recent study examined the five major allowable categories of community benefit: charity care, Medicaid shortfall (the difference between the cost of care for Medicaid patients in the institution and Medicaid's payments), unreimbursed means-tested patient care services, unreimbursed education costs for medical trainees, and unfunded research performed.[23]

The individual and total amounts were compared among three types of not-for-profit hospitals: secular, Catholic, and other church-operated hospitals. Secular hospitals provided 6.1%, Catholic hospitals 7.5%, and other church-operated hospitals 9.4% of their expenditures in total community benefit.[23]

Thirty-eight percent of Catholic hospitals' community benefit was the shortfall in Medicaid payments. Some researchers and states do not consider this in community benefit calculations, as it may be covered by other revenue sources.[23,24] Other church-operated hospitals provided a significantly higher percentage of their expenses as charity care than did Catholic hospitals: 5.2% versus 3.9%, respectively.[23] Excluding Medicaid shortfall, other church-operated hospitals provided $84,200 per bed as community benefit compared to $57,500 per bed provided by Catholic hospitals and $50,180 per bed by secular not-for-profit hospitals.[23]

One might expect Catholic hospitals to stand out in providing community benefit, given that they have an ERD mandate to care for the poor (Chapter 4), yet they fall behind the other church-operated hospitals. However, religiously sponsored not-for-profit hospitals, including Catholic facilities, are making a greater commitment than secular not-for-profit hospitals.

All not-for-profit hospitals receive the same tax benefits, but within and across groups, there is considerable variability in what they give back in community benefits. Also, others have pointed out that not-for-profit hospitals in an area of highly valued real estate receive greater value from their property tax than a similar hospital located in a poor area — quite the opposite of what would seem desirable.[25] Moreover, quite surprisingly, some studies have shown that for-profit hospitals that don't receive these tax-exemptions and do pay taxes provide more charity care.[26]

The Lown Institute Hospital Index specifically examines hospitals' and systems' community benefit contributions (Table 8.1). It excludes Medicaid shortfall and unfunded research and education, which is permitted by the IRS in the calculation of community benefit, as it is not possible to assess how much of these categories is covered by other sources of revenue[27] None of the large Catholic systems ranked in the top 100 systems in the provision of community benefit.[21]

Another way to consider community benefit is to compare the financial value of the tax-exemptions received to the community benefit that the hospitals provide. The recent study from the Kaiser Family Foundation calculated that the charity care provided by the not-for-profit hospitals in 2020 was $16 billion, considerably less than their $28 billion in tax benefits.[22]

The Lown Institute has calculated tax benefit and community benefit for not-for-profit hospitals and health systems, using 5.9% of expenses as the estimated tax-exemption and community benefit as defined above. If the tax exemption amount exceeds the amount of community benefit provided, this is labelled a fair share deficit. Seventy-seven percent of all not-for-profit hospitals have a fair share deficit.[28] All six of the large Catholic system have fair share deficits ranging from $142 million for SSM to $911 million for CommonSpirit (personal communication Judith Garber Lown Institute) (Table 8.2). These estimates were able to include most, but not all the hospitals in a given systems, so it could either slightly under-or over-estimate the fair share deficit.

TABLE 8.2. Fair Share Deficit

System	Hospitals Included	Year	Deficit
Ascension	83	2020	$407,763,814
Bon Secours MH	29	2019	$284,599,989
CommonSpirit	102	2020	$911,211,345
Providence	42	2019	$771,896,150
Trinity	61	2020	$616,718,040
SSM	19	2020	$141,935,172

Source: Fair Share Deficit analysis was conducted by Judith Garber at the Lown Institute using the most recent year of comprehensive tax data for each system as of March 2023. For each system, the number of unique tax IDs used is as follows: Ascension 60, Bon Secours Mercy Health 9, Common Spirit 56, Providence 15, SSM Health 12, Trinity 48.

The imbalance between taxes that local, state, and federal governments are losing and the benefits to communities and the country is gaining attention not only from researchers and policymakers, but also from communities and government. In February 2023, a court in Pennsylvania ruled that a not-for-profit healthcare system's hospitals were not eligible for property tax exemptions. This ruling resulted from suits filed by four school districts, triggered in part by the healthcare system's insufficient free care and executive compensation methods and amounts.[29]

At least four states recently updated community benefit criteria and/or reporting.[30] Oregon has set a floor for community benefit spending for tax-exempt hospitals.[30] On April 26, 2023 the House Ways and Means Committee held a hearing on tax-exempt hospitals and community benefit standards to hear the data and perspectives on the issue.

FINANCIAL PROFILES

At the beginning of Jesus' public teaching, he was clear about focusing on material goods: "*...where your treasure is there will your heart be also (Matthew 6: 21)*. Being well-schooled in Jesus' words, Mother Cabrini warned of the dangers of prosperity saying, "*We must beware of two temptations, that of failure and that of success; and often prosperity will be more dangerous than adversity (Chapter 3).*"[31]

ERD's Part 1, Directives 3, 6, and 7 are relevant to a discussion of Catholic healthcare's financial state (Chapter 4).[32] These require that Catholic healthcare institutions have primary concern for the poor, are good stewards of their resources, and treat their employees fairly, including providing just compensation. These issues are foundational components of Catholic Social Teaching (Chapter 4).

Examination of the most recently published financial reports for the large Catholic systems revealed that they have accumulated enormous wealth — all in the billions of dollars, with CommonSpirit topping the charts at $50.3 billion (Table 8.3).[3] The 2021–2022 Modern Healthcare reports of the largest healthcare systems by operating revenue revealed that CommonSpirit, Providence, Ascension, Trinity Health, Bon Secours Mercy Health, and SSM (fell below the top 25 in corrected version) were in the top twenty-five of all healthcare systems.[33]

All had operating revenues in the billions, with CommonSpirit topping the list at over $30 billion (Table 8.3)[33] All of these systems were on a par with the largest secular not-for-profit and for-profit health systems; only Kaiser Foundation Health Plan and Hospitals and HCA Healthcare had larger operating revenue than the top three Catholic health systems.[33]

Over and above this operating revenue, their IRS 990 forms revealed that they all had substantial investment income. In fact, Bon Secours Mercy Health has a private equity team[2] and Providence and Ascension have their own venture capital funds, with Ascension's totaling $1 billion.[34] This venture capital activity prompted a detailed investigative report by STAT News in 2021.[34] The report was the result of interviews with "*...academic experts, financial analysts, accountants, and community

TABLE 8.3. Financial Profiles of Catholic Healthcare Systems

System	Total Assets[1]	Operating Revenue[2]
Ascension	$44.1B	$25.26B
Bon Secours MH	$16.4B	$9.96B
CommonSpirit	$50.3B	$30.13B
Providence	$28.9B	$25.68B
SSM Health	$10.6B	$8.2B[3]
Trinity Health	$31.1B	$18.83B

1. Data accessed July 1, 2023 from most recent audited financial statement. Ascension, Trinity Health, CommonSpirit are through June 30, 2022. Providence, SSM, Bon Secours MH are through December 31, 2022.
   Resources:
   https://about.ascension.org/about-us/community-investor-relations
   https://about.ascension.org/-/media/project/ascension/about/section-about/financials/2022/consolidated-ascension-financial-statements-q4-fy22.pdf
   https://bsmhealth.org/financial-information/
   https://emma.msrb.org/P21680823-P21293352-P21723462.pdf
   https://www.commonspirit.org/investor-resources . Note: This CommonSpirit link denotes it as the annual audited financial statement, however when the document is opened the title page says it is an Unaudited Annual Report.
   https://www.providence.org/about/financial-statements Note: The report is noted as a 'Continuing Disclosure Annual Report.'
   https://www.providence.org/-/media/project/psjh/providence/socal/files/about/financial-statements/2022_continuing_disclosure_annual_report_wsupp_info_and_audit.pdf?la=en&rev=33cd15ccc74a4bd6bb36af85f17382ce&hash=06BA927564330A22E8FA9F874B6D456E page 12
   https://www.trinity-health.org/about-us/facts-and-figures-financial-strength
   https://www.trinity-health.org/assets/documents/financials/trinity-health-fy22-financial-statements-long-form-final.pdf
   https://www.ssmhealth.com/resources/about/financials/reports
   https://www.ssmhealth.com/SSMHealth/media/Documents/about/financial-reports/annual-financials-21–22.pdf
2. Data from Modern Healthcare Dec 20, 2021 (Corrected version published March 7,2022)
3. SSM from Dec. 20, 2021 Modern Healthcare. SSM not in the top 25 by revenue in corrected version.

organizers and a review of more than 3500 pages of financial disclosures, lawsuits, and previously undisclosed internal financial documents."[34]

Some information from that publication is as follows:[34]

- Ascension partnered with TowerBrook Capital Partners, a global equity firm.[32] Eileen Applelbaum, co-director of the Center for Economic and Policy Research, stated *"I am not aware of any other major health provider or big health system that has gotten this involved in private equity."*[34] Together they invested $200 million in Accretive (now R1 RMC), a debt collection firm that had been previously delisted from the

New York Stock Exchange.[34] Ascension made the firm its only billing and debt collector. In part because of these actions, the debt collector grew its revenue from $117 million to $1.3 billion.[34] Ascension reaped substantial benefits from its R1 RMC investment, claiming a return of over $500 million.[34]

- The two key employees who left Ascension for roles in Ascension Capital, Ascension's venture capital arm, saw their income go from $7.4 million to $10.6 million and from $3.1 million to $10.9 million.[34]
- While Ascension was amassing an earthly treasure, there were concerns about cutting needed staff at some of its facilities (see above). Also, it closed an unprofitable facility, Providence Hospital in Washington, DC, and was planning cuts to St. Joseph's Hospital in Wisconsin.[34] Providence hospital was one of the only two hospitals in a poor section of the city, with 50% of its patients having Medicaid as their insurance coverage.[35] This closure was concerning on at least two counts: Ascension's stated mission and Ascension's potential contribution to Providence's problem.

  At a Washington DC City Council meeting where the closure was being addressed, a representative of Ascension affirmed, *"Our mission... has always been 'Following in Jesus' footsteps, we are committed to serving...especially those who are poor or struggling...."*[35] A reporter's assessment of that statement was, *"Jesus' footsteps never carried Him...to a large bank account."*[35]

  Part of Providence's financial difficulties may have been due to the $27.5 million management fee Ascension charged Providence for back-end management, and the additional fees for services from the private equity companies it owned.[34] While mother ships do charge fees for the services they provide to a system's hospital members, the DC Attorney General deemed it likely exorbitant, resulting in Ascension forgiving $130 million of Providence's debt.[34]
- Ascension leaders state that its goal is *"generating capital gains that can be reinvested to support Ascension's Mission to care for those who are poor and vulnerable."*[34]

The experts quoted in the STAT article concluded:

- *"If you want to imagine an activity at the opposite end of something charitable, you might as well focus on a company that makes money by squeezing blood from a stone* [referring to the collection company].*"*[34]
- *"...it is not clear how those investment incomes and returns are aligned with Ascension's charitable mission."*[34]

Key questions that should be asked in light of these data are "Should a Catholic healthcare system be in the debt collecting business?" "Should Catholic healthcare systems be invested in venture capital companies?" "Should the supervising bishops see these activities as compatible with of Part 1 of the ERDs?"

In part as a result of the STAT article and Ascension's intention to cut services at its Wisconsin hospital, Senator Tammy Baldwin, one of Wisconsin's U.S. Senators, sent a detailed letter to Joseph Impicciche, Ascension CEO, stating, "*As a nonprofit, tax-exempt health system, Ascension is required ...solely to serve a public, rather than a private interest. Despite these requirements, Ascension has significant for-profit investment activities that dwarf what the system provides in annual charity care.*[36] Senator Baldwin asked to be provided with numerous documents to explain Ascension's actions. As of June 2023, I have been unable to obtain Impicciche's response to Senator Baldwin.

The federal government has contributed to the problem that Ascension demonstrates in a variety of ways, not the least of which is allowing hospitals that are a big business in America to have not-for-profit status in return for community benefits. While the broad categories that are acceptable for community benefit have been delineated and the healthcare facilities must report those contributions to the IRS, no threshold for community benefit has been set. Hence, there is enormous variability in community benefits that not-for-profit hospitals provide.[23] Moreover, the old adage "*Trust but verify*" is not in play when it comes to not-for-profit community benefits.

Another surprising way in which the government seems to have contributed is the 1998 IRS ruling that created a "*pathway for non-profit hospitals to profit tax-free from partnerships with for-profit companies.*"[34,37] There are a number of requirements in the IRS ruling for these relationships, including: [37]

- The relationship operates "*in a manner that furthers charitable purposes by promoting the health of a broad cross section of the community.*"
- "*None of the officers, directors, or key employees of the nonprofit who were involved in decision making or the negotiations involving the formation of the LLC were promised employment or any other inducement by the for-profit, the LLC, or their related entities.*"

One wonders if the IRS carefully examines all of these relationships to determine if they fulfill these requirements.

The women religious begged for pennies and dollars wherever they could. The large Catholic systems still solicit funds from patients and the public, but they seem to have "upped the ask." The systems and the individual hospitals both have foundations and solicit donor support. CommonSpirit's Foundation reports that it has over 80 different foundations and that it has raised $1.3 billion in five years, of which $300 million was received in 2022.[38]

Ascension has at least 52 foundations in 14 states and the District of Columbia — the total value of which is not clear.[39] However, the *Urban Milwaukee* paper reported that the total assets of the foundations of the six Ascension hospitals in Wisconsin was $148 million.[39]

Providence St. Joseph's system has 40 foundations in seven states and raised over $359 million in 2022.[40] Bon Secours Mercy Health has 12 foundations in five states, with assets of more than $370 million in 2020, raising approximately $92.5 million in the first seven months of 2022.[41,42] SSM has a foundation received over $11 million in revenue in 2021.[43] Trinity Health appears to have a number of foundations, but information on the Trinity Health System Foundation is not easily found.

Of course, virtually all hospitals and systems have foundations, and they serve good purposes for patients and the community. Similarly, all of these foundations report giving grants and supporting a range of services in their communities. As with other hospital foundations, many of the expenditures appear to be for services and construction for their own systems. Providing the information on these foundations is only to underscore that these systems have amassed large amounts of money.

EXECUTIVES VS EMPLOYEES

The American bishops' 1986 letter on *Economic Justice for All* stated, "*The concentration of privilege that exists today results far more from institutional relationships that distribute power and wealth inequitably… These institutional patterns must be examined and revised….*"[44]

While that statement was referring primarily to the societal relationships of institutions, it has important relevance for the distribution of wealth within Catholic institutions. In 2014, Pope Francis, in a Twitter message, placed a heavy judgment on inequality, saying, "*Inequality is the root of social evil.*"[45] Therefore, we should expect to see a just distribution of resources reflected in the wages of employees in Catholic healthcare systems.

Two related measurements of that equitable distribution are executive compensation and the relationship between the compensation of those executives and other employees, especially the lowest paid employees. The CEO compensation at SSM and Trinity is about $2 million, which is close to the median total cash compensation for large systems.[46] The other four systems have compensation for the CEO near to or more than $8 million annually; Bon Secours Mercy tops the charts at $ 12.7 million (Table 8.4).

For most people, those numbers are not comprehensible, given that real median earnings of all U.S. workers aged 15 and over is $41,535.[47] A way to make it more comprehensible is to compare those CEOs' salaries to a housekeeper, one of the lowest paid employees, and to a registered nurse, a key provider in healthcare (Table 8.4). Another perspective is to consider the base salary and incentive compensation of the key executives listed on IRS 990 and calculate how many housekeepers and registered nurses could be hired with that amount of money (Table 8.4).

While salaries vary between individual hospitals for housekeepers based on a number of factors, including the hospital's location, the average salary nationally for housekeepers in hospitals is $29,744.[48] Similarly, while registered nurses' salaries vary based on location of the hospital and the type of work the nurse is performing, the median salary for a registered nurse is $81,220.[49] The calculation is simply to create some understandable comparisons for the magnitude of the executive salaries in the Catholic healthcare systems.

The gap between executives and others in the workforce reflects the commitment to equity. For Bon Secours Mercy Health, the CEO's compensation is 428 times that of a housekeeper's salary and 157 times that of a registered nurse's salary. Ascension tops the chart for the compensation of its top executive team with the five highest paid Ascension employees receiving $26.9 million a year which could pay for 903 housekeepers or 331 nurses (Table 8.4). This information raises the question, "Is the compensation of executives and the relationship to key components of the workforce in line with Catholic Social Teaching?" (see Chapter 4).

In 2018, Michael Sean Winters, a reporter for the *National Catholic Reporter*, interviewed Ascension's chief ethicist who told him that all senior executives in the organization *"receive on-going formation that includes a heavy dose of Catholic social teaching."*[35] Later that same day, Winters asked the then-CEO of Ascension Health how the executive salaries reflected Pope Francis' statement on inequality. Her response was, *"I am not going to get into that conversation."*[35] Exorbitant executive salaries were part of the reason the tax-exempt status was removed from four not-for-profit hospitals (non-Catholic) in Pennsylvania (See above).[29]

TABLE 8.4. Compensation Comparisons in Catholic Healthcare Systems

System	CEO Compensation[1]	Times Housekeeper[2]	Times Reg Nurse[3]	Total Top 5 Execs[1]	N of HK[4]	N of RN[5]
Ascension	$12.36M	416	152	$26.9M	903	331
Bon Secours*	$12.73M	428	157	$18.3M	616	226
CommonSpirit	$7.94M	267	98	$24.4M	821	301
Providence	$8.25M	277	102	$15.5M	521	191
SSM	$2.13M	72	26	$6.1M	206	75
Trinity	$2.42M	81	30	$8.0M	270	99

1. Data from the most recently filed IRS 990* Schedule J, Part II, (B) Breakdown of W-2 and/or 1099-MISC compensation column (i) Base Compensation and column (ii) Bonus & incentive Compensation; top five executive compensation equals total (i) Base Compensation and (ii) Bonus & incentive Compensation for the top five total compensation. All compensation includes reported compensation for both row (i) organization and row (ii) related organization.
2. This is the number of multiples the CEO's compensation (total base plus bonus & incentive compensation) is of the average for a healthcare housekeeper of $29,744 data from ZipRecruiter accessed August 11, 2023
3. This is the number of multiples the CEO's compensation (total base plus bonus & incentive compensation) is of the median salary for a registered nurse of $81,220 data from Bureau of Labor Statistics accessed March 7, 2023.
4. This is the number of housekeepers who could be hired at the average salary with the base plus bonus and incentive compensation of the top five executives
5. This is the number of registered nurses who could be hired at the median salary with the base plus bonus and incentive compensation of the top five executives
*Bon Secours refers to Bon Secours Mercy Health

Much data about the workforce that are not available would be useful in assessing the Catholic healthcare system's commitment to equity and Catholic Social Teaching. These data include:

- The racial and ethnic distribution of the workforce at all levels of the hierarchical structure.
- The percentage of the workforce, including contract workers, who are making salaries below the living wage.
- Whether there is pay equity across race and gender.
- Whether there is paid leave for all employees, including contract workers.
- Whether there is affordable health insurance coverage for all employees, including contract workers.

The Catholic healthcare systems could and should be leaders in providing these employee supports and in transparently reporting them. They should lead the healthcare sector in zealous commitment to equity for all their employees. Their boards and the overseeing bishops should require this.

PATIENT CARE

While financial behavior and care of the poor are central in evaluating whether Catholic healthcare is true to its theological and historical roots, the quality of patient care is a prime measure of any healthcare system. Although there are significant concerns related to the care that is prohibited and not provided to patients who come through their doors (Chapters 4 and 5), the care that is provided should be of high quality and the systems should not be performing services that are deemed to be of low value.

Capturing the quality of care is challenging, but a number of organizations use a cadre of measures to assess it. The Lown Institute Hospital Index includes a component for patient outcomes that incorporates hospital mortality, 30- and 90-day mortality, and 7- and 30-day readmission for Medicare fee-for-service and Medicare Advantage patients.

Of the Catholic healthcare systems, four ranked in the top 100 (top tertile): Providence #28, CommonSpirit #69, Trinity #89, and Bon Secours Mercy Health #90 (Table 8.1).[21] The Lown Institute Hospital Index also measures the extent to which hospitals and systems avoid 12 tests or procedures that are considered to be ineffective or of low value.[21] Of the large Catholic systems, only Providence ranked in the top 100 for avoiding overuse, coming in at 100. (Table 8.1).[21]

Another important aspect of quality is patient safety. The Leapfrog Group and Lown both report on this measure. The Leapfrog gives individual hospitals safety grades of A through F, utilizing *"twenty-two national patient safety measures from the Centers for Medicare & Medicaid Services (CMS), the Leapfrog Hospital Survey, and information from other supplemental data sources."*[50] The Leapfrog Group grades about 3,000 general acute-care hospitals, excluding critical access hospitals, twice annually. In 2020, 896 of the 2700 hospitals (33%) received an A grade for patient safety, (Personal communication, Kush Banerjee, Leapfrog).

Of the 392 Catholic hospitals on the 2020 AHA hospital survey (critical access excluded), 119 received a grade of A in Leapfrog (30%), (Personal communication, Kush Banerjee, Leapfrog).

The Lown Institute Hospital Index ranks hospitals and systems from best to worst using data from CMS Care, the CMS composite measure of 10 indicators of patient safety, and five hospital-acquired infection measures. The Lown Index ranked two of the Catholic hospital systems in the top 100: Providence (#69) and Ascension (#99).[21]

CONCLUSION

The evolution in Catholic healthcare in America from its origins in the 1800s and early 1900s has been a success story by business standards. The systems have become vast, rich, and powerful. The American bishops and many Catholics might say it has been a success in adhering to its deepest theological beliefs by avoiding care that it deems immoral, and in helping create the legal environment in which to freely exercise those beliefs in healthcare.

That would be true. In doing so, these healthcare institutions seem to imply they follow a higher ethical standard. But that raises other questions. Do these institutions behave just as other large healthcare entities in their business practices? Should Catholic healthcare have a higher bar? Is their commitment to the poor and most vulnerable reflected in all their policies and behaviors? Do they demonstrate fidelity to their stated mission? Are they walking in the footsteps of Jesus' healing ministry? How does the inequity within their institutions and their corporate wealth align with the long history of Catholic Social Teaching?

Catholic healthcare has stored much wealth in their earthly treasure chests. Is that where their hearts now lie?

CHAPTER 9

Walking the Old Path and Building New Roads

Do to others whatever you would have them do to you.
Jesus, Matthew 7:12

Chapters 1 through 8 of this book are a journey from ancient times to today. The journey reveals the Judaic-Christian theology that created a moral imperative to heal the sick, presents Jesus' ministry of healing, and details the unwavering commitment of Catholic religious women to follow that example and create institutions delivering on that commitment.

The journey moves from small hospitals built in areas of need run by those vowing poverty to large corporations built to capture market share and seemingly committed to profit. The journey paints the individual, organizational, and societal complexities between the competing rights of religious freedom to act as one believes and that freedom constraining the rights of the majority who do not share that religion; between individual conscience and organizational conscience; between patient autonomy and organizational rules; between physicians' oath and employment requirements; between Catholic institutions advocating publicly for society to embrace their views on life and death and lack of transparency about prohibitions emanating from those views within their healthcare institutions.

The journey details the reach of Catholic healthcare institutions across 46 states with hospitals, clinics, free-standing emergency departments, urgent care centers, and health plans, and with non-Catholic healthcare institutions. This vast network provides a substantial volume of high-quality care to millions of Americans in rural areas and urban centers.

This is a good to be valued. However, Catholic healthcare, like every human organization, is not without its limitations and flaws. These limits and flaws need to be clearly seen by all who use the healthcare system and those who oversee it in the Church and in government. Therefore, this written journey is intended both to inspire us and to raise concerns and critical questions.

But the book cannot conclude by showing only what is good and posing the hard questions. There needs to be some attempt to define the next steps in the journey. We need to ask what should change, what can enable that change, and who can make those changes. The answer to those questions leads us backward to old beaten paths and forward to new, yet unbuilt roads.

Some details for those old roads and new paths are presented below. Some are for the Catholic Church, and some are specifically for Catholic healthcare institutions. Others are for all religious institutions. Some reach to all not-for-profit healthcare entities. Some steps seem feasible, and some may be only aspirations. But all change is a process and a journey that starts with the first step. Former Colorado Governor Richard Lamm laid out the sequence by which any significant change happens:

Step 1: No talk, no do

This is the period when the problem is not even known and certainly not discussed. We have been at this place for a long time with regard to the current issues in Catholic healthcare in America. No problem can be addressed if it has not been named or if only a few lone voices have surfaced it.

Step 2: Talk, no do

This is a period when many voices raise the issue and push the need for action. More voices are now bringing to the American public the issues raised by Catholic healthcare. More constructive dialogue must occur. This will not be easy at a time when society has moved away from civil, problem-solving discourse.

Step 3: Do, no talk

This is the phase of action when we stop talking about the issues and actually fix them. This is where we must head. But we must also realize that solutions themselves take time and not every problem will be solved today, or tomorrow, or even perhaps, in our lifetime.

THE CHURCH AND CHANGE

As is often the case with individuals, one's greatest strength can also be their greatest weakness, and so it may also be with the Catholic Church.

It changes positions very slowly, often taking decades or even centuries. This lets its believers stand on solid ground. They know that a long-held practice or belief will not change with the first winds of dissent. On the other hand, new knowledge, greater understanding, and societal change can take a long time to translate into new views and behavior, but change can happen.

It took almost 400 years of saying Mass in Latin before it was said in the language of the people, but it did happen. The Church moved from persecuting Galileo for the heresy of saying the earth revolved around the sun to allowing books endorsing the fact — although it took more than 100 years.

Some beliefs and teachings are so foundational to the faith that it is unlikely they could ever change and be Catholicism. But perhaps, some views that create the healthcare prohibitions of today can change with new knowledge and time.

So, the question has two parts: (1) Can some of those long and deeply held beliefs help Catholic healthcare institutions walk back to their admirable and noble past, and (2) Can there be space for healthcare institutions to provide some now-prohibited healthcare when new knowledge is acquired? These are the questions that hang over Catholic healthcare in America.

The Hierarchy

Given the strong hierarchical structure of the Catholic Church, a return to past commitments and any change in current views must start at the top with the pope. Pope Francis has been a vigorous supporter of the poor, the vulnerable, and immigrants. He has stood against the imbalance of power and wealth. In these areas he has been an example of Christ-like mercy. He has asked all Catholics, especially the hierarchy, to walk that same beaten path.

This should apply to Catholic healthcare institutions as well. They should be a model of an unmistakable commitment to the poor and of the just distribution of their wealth both within and outside their walls. Pope Francis has been less judgmental of others who may not align with Catholic beliefs. Again, he has urged the hierarchy to be less judgmental and more compassionate to those on the margin, those who face many trials, and those who do not share Catholic beliefs.

I have not been formally schooled in theology or in the teachings of the Church on the many issues of faith and morals. Even if I were, it would be inappropriate for me to suggest what the pope should do. But I can applaud the commitments he has already made and the examples that he gives. Thus, I will only pose questions for consideration by those with this knowledge, understanding, and responsibility.

The pope has called for greater dialogue within the whole community of the Catholic Church as demonstrated by the synods that are being held in Rome in 2023 and 2024 (see Chapter 4).

- Can this dialogue in America include voices of many lay and religious women whose lived experience differs from that of the male hierarchy?
- Can this dialogue be an opening of discussion with the theologians and Catholics in the body of the Church who have had a dissenting opinion on a range of issues related to healthcare?
- Can this dialogue include a broad swath of scientists and physicians? Given the theological basis and centuries of teaching against abortion and medical aid-in-dying, it seems dialogue could not change those positions. However, many other aspects of healthcare that relate to reproduction, sexuality, and dying may not be set in stone.
- Can it be possible to have clarity on allowing a pregnancy to be terminated if there is a non-viable fetus in the circumstance of a miscarriage or ectopic pregnancy?
- Can the Church rethink the mantra that a beating heart is a line in the sand? Is this linked to some ancient idea that the heart is the seat of the soul? Or is it a line in the sand only because it is easy to measure? If the answer is "Yes" to those two questions, perhaps that line can be reconsidered.
- Can the assertion that a rape victim can receive emergency contraception, as is stated in the ERDs (Chapter 4) be underscored so that there is not variability in this care across Catholic healthcare institutions?
- Can the use of artificial contraception in marriage be left to the conscience of couples, as has been endorsed by some theologians? If intercourse is allowed when a woman is not ovulating or is post-menopausal, why can't that state of non-ovulation occur with the drugs that science has enabled?
- Can the Church be open to the idea that marital intercourse brings more to a marriage than procreation?
- Is it possible to allow artificial insemination if the husband's sperm is used?

- Can the Church rethink the position that the provision of artificial nutrition is indeed part of a natural death?
- Will it be possible to rethink the nature of gender as new knowledge is obtained?

Some will say these questions have long been decided by those with deep knowledge and understanding of Catholic beliefs. But when so many practicing Catholics and even some theologians are asking these questions, shouldn't those decisions be discussed anew with more people at the table?

Unlike the need to only raise questions on issues that pertain to faith and morals, the information presented in the preceding chapters, and my own experience as a physician leader, permit me to put forth a series of concrete suggestions to the American bishops on Catholic healthcare.

Given that the bishops have asserted their supervisory role over Catholic healthcare institutions, they must step up in new ways to exert their oversight of Catholic healthcare in dimensions that go beyond sex, reproduction, and death.

The American bishops are to be applauded for emphasizing in Part 1 of the ERDs the central role of care for the poor and fair treatment of employees, including just compensation. They must enforce compliance with this obligation with the same fervor that they have for other aspects of the ERDs.

Several years ago, I informed a previous Archbishop of Denver about behavior of a Catholic healthcare system which I believed was in stark contrast to the obligation to care for the poor. His reply was that he could only act in cases violating the ERDs. Yet, this is the first obligation of ERDs:

> *"Catholic healthcare should distinguish itself by service to and advocacy for those people whose social condition puts them at the margins of our society and makes them particularly vulnerable to discrimination: the poor, the uninsured, and the underinsured…"* (see Chapter 4).

The United States Council of Catholic Bishops should issue a clear statement to all Catholic healthcare institutions and to all Americans that they are zealously committed to enforcing this part of the ERDs.

To walk the talk, they need to require the following from every Catholic healthcare institution regarding the care of the poor, the just use of their resources, and their advocacy:

- Maintenance of an open-door policy for all individuals in the same way as do the traditional safety net healthcare institutions.
- Establishment of robust, completely transparent, and accessible financial aid for patients below 400% of the federal poverty level.
- Prohibition of policies that permit turning patients over to collection agencies, selling patient debt, taking legal action against patients for debt, and denying non-emergency care for patients with debt.
- Guarantees that all employees, including contract employees, are paid a living wage, and are provided with healthcare, parental leave, and paid time off.
- A cap for executive salaries in terms of actual dollar amount and percentage by which it can exceed that of the lowest paid employees, as well as complete transparency about salaries and total compensation of all the executives of hospitals and systems.
- Provision that direct community benefit contributions equal or exceed the tax benefits and reflect meaningful partnerships with the specific communities they serve regarding those community benefits.
- Requirement that closing a healthcare facility within a minority-serving or underserved area is approved by the bishop of that diocese.
- Creation of guidelines for the institution's investment policies and levels of reserves that comport with their primary social mission.
- Requirement that boards agree to and operationalize these expectations.

The American bishops have created and enforced the ERDs in part to create a moral example. Therefore, they must be transparent about the Church's beliefs and how those beliefs impact patient care. They must affirm the following:

- Every Catholic healthcare institution must state on its landing page that it is a Catholic institution and abides by the ERDs.
- There must be a link on the landing page to the ERDs in a format and language that is accessible to all patients.
- Every Catholic healthcare institution must enumerate all procedures prohibited by the ERDs in a list linked to its landing page and to its relevant consent forms.

The American bishops have considered changes to Part 3 of the ERDs, which defines the Professional-Patient Relationship at their regular June 2023 meeting (Chapter 5). Their focus is on gender-affirming care (Chapter 5). They should be encouraged to continue their examination to permit greater alignment of physicians with their professional oath and code of ethics. They should establish a dialogue with a range of physician groups to re-examine the components that prevent physicians from engaging in shared decision-making with their patients and from referring patients to organizations that provide care that is medically appropriate and that the patient desires, but is prohibited in the Catholic healthcare institution in which the physicians practice.

Finally, as Part 1 of the ERDs dictates, the American bishops must be a forceful voice for policies that improve the social condition of the poor and those on the margin, raising their voices for a living wage, paid time off, access to high-quality care for all mothers and children, universal healthcare, fair housing practices, and similar issues.

American healthcare needs transformation in many dimensions. With these actions, the bishops would establish Catholic healthcare institutions as a worthy example for American healthcare in these specific areas.

Women Religious Congregations

Although the number of women religious has dwindled and those who remain are often elderly, the previous generation of women in those communities laid the foundations for the current large healthcare systems and their voice and values must still be heard today.

The congregations could and should examine the Catholic healthcare systems in light of the goals, mission, and care of their founders and ask if these systems now truly honor that legacy, particularly in care of the poor and avoidance of greed. If the healthcare systems do not, their boards should be engaged in conversations that return the systems to their historic mission.

Organizations of Catholic women religious and individual women religious, who have been unrelenting advocates for social justice, should carefully examine the behaviors of Catholic healthcare institutions regarding mission fidelity and Catholic Social Teaching.

The Body of the Church

All the members of the Church are considered essential to the body of the Church and to its existence and function (Chapter 4). Although there is not unanimity among American Catholics on a range of issues, particularly around reproductive care, we should be able to agree on many aspects of Jesus' examples of compassion and healing.

Therefore, every Catholic should be aware of Catholic healthcare's role in American healthcare and how this care is operationalized. Catholics should advocate for it to truly provide God's healing care to everyone. They should expect transparency from Catholic healthcare institutions. All Catholics need to be engaged in dialogue about how to find the line between the Catholic hospitals' commitment to their beliefs and every patient's own conscience and autonomy.

GOVERNMENT

Rules of Conscience

The government in all its branches has the unenviable task of balancing the two components of the First Amendment. It seems unlikely that any of the rules of conscience that currently exist for individuals or organizations will be changed to require individuals or religious healthcare facilities or providers to perform procedures that they deem immoral. However, it should be expected and required that patients understand the care limitations that exist in these institutions.

Transparency should not just be a goal, but a requirement. Just as the federal government has required that hospitals provide price transparency and have readily available and useable information on prices of procedures, it should require transparency of religious affiliation and readily available and easily useable information on care that will not be provided based on religious beliefs.

Linking religious affiliation with care that is not provided is important for two reasons. First, there are thousands of procedures and few, if any, healthcare systems do them all for a variety of reasons. Therefore, it would not be feasible for every hospital to list every procedure it does not perform. Secondly, as discussed in Chapter 5, patients often do not know if a hospital is religiously affiliated. If they do know, they do not expect care limitations based on that affiliation. This requirement should apply not only to Catholic hospitals but to all religiously affiliated hospitals that prohibit some types of care.

Providing price transparency has been challenging because of the enormous numbers of procedures and the variability in what a patient might consider a single procedure. It will be much easier to provide the list of prohibited procedures.

While ideally this would be a federal requirement just as is price transparency, individual states should enact such requirements if the federal government does not. In fact, some states have done so. This would be especially important in the states with the highest percentage of Catholic healthcare institutions. This information should be on website landing pages with clear links to the lists. The information should also be in consent forms, particularly for treatment and admissions in areas most likely to be affected, such as reproductive and obstetrical care. Colorado has recently taken steps in this direction and other states should follow. Truly informed consent and shared decision making must be assured.

The federal government should re-examine religiously based care limitations in sole community providers, critical access hospitals, and in hospitals that are in a geographic area in which all the hospitals have the same religious prohibitions.

On the one hand, requiring these hospitals to provide the range of medically appropriate care that they have the technical and professional capacity to provide would improve patient care and guarantee equal access for care to patients with limited or no provider choice. However, such a requirement might lead Catholic facilities to abandon certain services such as obstetric care or close these hospitals, leaving patients with no care. This will be difficult terrain to traverse, but it should not be ignored, as it can have profound effects on the patients who have no other readily available source of care.

The federal and state governments must assess the consequences of the prohibitions of certain procedures or types of care in Catholic healthcare institutions for patients with government healthcare coverage, especially Medicaid and the subsidized Marketplace Health Insurance plans.

Given Medicaid's critical role in care for the poor and in maternity and reproductive care for a high percentage of women, the government must assess and ensure that these patients are reliably informed about religiously based limitations of care in any healthcare facility that accepts Medicaid. These patients must have easy referral and access to covered services that may not be provided at a specific healthcare institution based on religious beliefs.

Again, ideally this would be a responsibility of federal agencies. However, Medicaid is a state-federal partnership, and those states in which a substantial amount of obstetrical care occurs in Catholic hospitals should establish this requirement and provide oversight.

While there is less information on Catholic healthcare's impact on end-of-life care than on the range of reproductive care, this is an area that the Church regulates. Hence, Medicare recipients, in particular, should be aware of the Catholic ownership and the end-of-life care that can be provided, is required, or prohibited.

Given the power that insurance companies have in selecting the hospitals that are in-network, these entities should be required to be transparent about their in-network providers whose care is limited by the ERDs or other religious prohibitions. The state government agencies that oversee insurance companies should require and enforce this provision.

Another area in which religiously based prohibited care becomes relevant is when a secular hospital merges with or is acquired by a Catholic system. Changes in available care should be completely transparent to the affected communities. Agencies of the state government that oversee such mergers and acquisitions should require this.

Tax Exemptions

The "Grand Bargain" of tax exemption in return for providing valuable healthcare to a community began in the Roman Empire with the Catholic Church. Is this still a reasonable quid pro quo 2000 years later, not just for Catholic hospitals but for all not-for profit hospitals? Two thousand years ago, much healthcare was truly charity care. Today healthcare, including "not-for-profit" healthcare, is a big business, as reflected in its executive salaries, its bottom lines, its cash reserves, and its capital investments. Moreover, the value of the tax-exemption has grown as the value of land, buildings and investment income has grown.

The enormous value of tax exemptions for not-for-profit hospitals, and the failure of their community benefit to reflect this value, makes this a critical question. In addition, the substantial variability among the not-for-profit hospitals and healthcare systems, all of which get the same tax benefits, raises other issues of fairness.

A first step in leveling the playing field in this area would be to define more precisely what qualifies as a community benefit. Some organizations and some states do not include medical training and research in that category. If these continue to be included, the actual value of these activities must be better defined, as they both have other tax dollars supporting them as well as benefits that accrue to the entities providing them.

Similarly, the large contributions of Medicaid shortfall to community benefits have been questioned and disallowed in some calculations. This requires further assessment, including whether some of that shortfall is covered by other revenues, including disproportionate share payments or higher cost and/or larger amounts of revenue from commercial insurance.

There needs to be recognition that the word "community" in "community benefit" implies that the community affected should be engaged in some meaningful way in what is provided.

A variety of proposals presented regarding tax-exemption, community benefit, and their relationship were detailed in the 2023 Kaiser Family Foundation study on tax exemption (see Chapter 8). These include:

- Requirements for hospitals to provide charity care to patients below a specified level of income.
- Requirements that a specified percentage of operating revenue be charity care.
- Establishment of a floor-and-trade system in which hospitals that do not meet the required floor provide funding to hospitals that exceed it.
- Replacement of tax-exemption with a government subsidy based on specified amounts of community benefit.

Of course, the option exists to abandon tax exemption for not-for-profit hospitals completely, an unlikely step.

The IRS should re-examine its 1998 ruling that enabled non-profit hospitals to profit tax-free from partnerships with for-profit companies (Chapter 8).

PROFESSIONAL ORGANIZATIONS

Some professional organizations and non-governmental regulatory bodies need to examine their relationship to Catholic healthcare organizations. The AMA, state, and county medical associations should examine the implications of the restrictions of the ERDs on employment and medical staff privileges on physician autonomy, and the physicians' professed oath to put the patients' needs above their own. This will require publicly acknowledging these implications and engaging in dialogue with the organizations, and most probably, the American bishops.

The training healthcare professionals receive is clearly dependent upon the environment in which that training occurs, and their adequate exposure to and participation in the range of care they will be expected to provide to patients. This applies especially to physicians, nurse practitioners, physician assistants and nurses. The schools which train these professionals and the accrediting bodies for that training must pay specific attention to the limitations of training that occurs in Catholic hospitals.

CONCLUSION

Regardless of the external rules imposed by bishops, or actions by women religious congregations, or government or professional organizations, meaningful change will occur only if the Catholic healthcare organizations' boards and their CEOs and executives believe and act in ways that return them to their roots.

No magic wand exists to create this return of Catholic healthcare to its old path or facilitate its building new roads. Even agreement that these steps are worthy ones by those with the power and those who use the system would be transformational. If the Catholic healthcare institutions alone adopted the suggestions detailed above, this would an enormous step forward, providing an example for others. American healthcare and society would be better and stronger.

We can hope for, work for, and pray that the Catholic Church and its hospitals begin leading the way back to the future, truly reflecting that the Church and its hospitals are a marriage made in heaven.

REFERENCES

Chapter 1: The Foundations of Healing

1. Ferngren GB. *Medicine and Health Care in Early Christianity*. Baltimore, MD: Johns Hopkins University Press, 2016.
2. Smith H. *The World's Religions: Our Great Wisdom Traditions*. New York: Perfect Bound HarperCollins Publishers, 1991.
3. Anderson GA. *Charity: The Place of the Poor in the Biblical Tradition*. New Haven, CT: Yale University Press, 2013.
4. Henriksen J, Sandnes, KO. *Jesus as Healer: A Gospel for the Body*. Grand Rapids, MI: William B. Eerdmans Publishing, 2016.
5. *Salvifici Doloris*. https://www.vatican.va/content/john-paul-ii/en/apost_letters/1984/documents/hf_jp-ii_apl_11021984_salvifici-doloris.html
6. Rohr R. Upending the Social Order. Daily Meditation. Center for Action and Contemplation. May 8, 2023. https://cac.org/daily-meditations/upending-the-social-order-2023-05-08/
7. Avalos H. *Health Care and the Rise of Christianity*. Peabody, MA: Hendrickson Publishers, 1999.
8. Ziegler TA. *Medieval Healthcare and the Rise of Charitable Institutions: The History of the Municipal Hospital*. New York: Springer Nature Publishing, 2018.
9. Crislip AT. *From Monastery to Hospital: Christian Monasticism and the Transformation of Health Care in Late Antiquity*. Ann Arbor, MI: University of Michigan Press, 2005.
10. St. Benedict. *Rule of Saint Benedict. (Kindle Edition)*. Translated by Boniface Verheyen. Christ the King Library, 2017.

Chapter 2: The Beginnings of Catholic Healthcare in America

1. Farren S. *A Call to Care: The Women Who Built Catholic Healthcare in America*. St. Louis, MO: Catholic Health Association of United States, 1996.
2. Fialka JJ. *Sisters: Catholic Nuns and the Making of America*. New York: St. Martin's Press, 2003.
3. McGuinness MM. *Called to Serve: A History of Nuns in America*. New York: New York University Press, 2013.
4. Kauffman CJ. *Meaning and Ministry: A Religious History of Catholic Health Care in the United States*. New York: The Crossroad Publishing Company, 1995
5. Carey P. Civil War Catholics. *First Things: A Monthly Journal of Religion and Public Life*. February 2020. https://www.firstthings.com/article/2020/02/civil-war-catholics.
6. U.S. National Park Service. Nuns of the Battlefield Memorial. National Mall and Memorial Parks. www.nps.gov/places/000/nuns-of-the-battlefield-memorial.htm.

7. Strickling L. *The Daughters of Charity and the Battle of Gettysburg.* Blog. Gettysburg National Military Park. August 22, 2019. https://npsgnmp.wordpress.com.
8. Stockman D. Research Shows Original Congregations of Sisters of Charity Owned Slaves. *Catholic Review.* February 15, 2022. https://catholicreview.org/research-shows-original-congregations-of-sisters-of-charity-owned-slaves.
9. Swarns RL. The Nuns Who Bought and Sold Human Beings. *New York Times,* August 2, 2019.
10. Herzog G, Norris MC. Letter from the Sisters of Charity Federation. February 7, 2022. https://sistersofcharityfederation.org/wp-content/uploads/2022/02/SC-Federation-Letter-Feb-7-2022.pdf.
11. Duriga J. Daniel Rudd: A Pioneering Leader in Black Catholic Journalism. *CRUX.* February 23, 2019. https://cruxnow.com/church-in-the-usa/2019/02/daniel-rudd-a-pioneering-leader-in-black-catholic-journalism.
12. St. Martin De Porres Hospital. Clio. https://theclio.com/entry/19235.
13. United States Conference of Catholic Bishops. *Open Wide Our Hearts: The Enduring Call to Love — A Pastoral Letter Against Racism.* Washington, DC: United States Conference on Catholic Bishops, November 2018. (©USCCB, Washington, DC. All rights reserved. Used by permission.) https://www.usccb.org/resources/open-wide-our-hearts-enduring-call-love-pastoral-letter-against-racism.
14. Lucia E. *Cornerstone: The Story of St. Vincent — Oregon's First Hospital.* Portland, OR: St. Vincent Medical Foundation, 1975.
15. Friedman E. Fulfilling the Sisters' Promise. The Heritage of Healthcare's Early Days. *Health Progress.* 1997;78(1):50–55.
16. Wall BM. "Definite Lines of Influence": Catholic Sisters and Nurse Training Schools, 1890–1920. *Nursing Research.* 2001;50(5):314–321.
17. Catholic Colleges Offering Nursing Schools. https://catholic-colleges.com/nursing.
18. Barthel J. *American Saint: The Life of Elizabeth Seton.* New York: Macmillan, 2014.
19. Wall BM. *American Catholic Hospitals: A Century of Changing Markets and Missions.* Princeton, NJ: Rutgers University Press, 2011.
20. Catholic Sisters' Letter in Support of Healthcare Reform Bill. Blog. *Network.* March 17, 2010. https://networklobby.org/20100317healthcare.

Chapter 3: Exemplary Mothers

1. Hanley ML, Bushnell OA. *A Song of Pilgrimage and Exile: The Life and Spirit of Mother Marianne of Molokai.* Chicago, IL: Franciscan Herald Press, 1980.
2. St. Marianne Cope. *Catholic News Agency.* https://www.catholicnewsagency.com/saint/st-marianne-cope-727.
3. Di Donato P. *Immigrant Saint: The Life of Mother Cabrini.* Auckland, NZ: Pickle Partners Publishing, 2017.

4. Missionary Sisters of the Sacred Heart of Jesus. Mother Cabrini. Missionary Sisters of the Sacred Heart of Jesus. https://www.mothercabrini.org/who-we-are/mother-cabrini.
5. Farren S. The Sisters Knew a Child Needs a Home. *Health Progress*. May-June 2011. https://www.chausa.org/docs/default-source/health-progress/the-sisters-knew---a-child-needs-a-home-pdf.
6. CNA Staff. Mother Cabrini's Order Celebrates 75th Anniversary of Her Canonization. *Catholic News Agency*. July 7, 2021. https://www.catholicnewsagency.com/news/248302/mother-cabrinis-order-celebrates-75th-anniversary-of-her-canonization.
7. Lucia E. *Cornerstone: The Formative Years of St. Vincent — Oregon's First Hospital*. Portland, OR: St. Vincent Medical Foundation, 1975.
8. Providence. Pioneer, Leader, Woman of Faith. Providence Archives. https://www.providence.org/about/providence-archives/history-online/mother-joseph-of-the-sacred-heart/pioneer.
9. Proceedings in the Rotunda of the United States Capital. Washington, DC, May 1, 1980.
10. Modern Healthcare. By the Numbers: Resource Guide 2021–2022. Modern Healthcare. December 20, 2021.
11. Day MAC. *A Woman for All Times: The Life of Mother Odilia (née Katharina Berger), Foundress of the Sisters of St. Mary of the Third Order of St. Francis*. St. Louis, MO: Sisters of St. Mary, 1980.
12. SSM Health. Our Heritage of Healing. Video. SSM Health. https://www.youtube.com/watch?v=Ci3n3Br_7w4.
13. Barthel J. *American Saint: The Life of Elizabeth Seton*. New York: St. Martin's Press, 2014.
14. Williamson E. Emmitsburg Nuns Keep Legacy of Charity Alive. *The Washington Post*. June 5, 2003.
15. Gettysburg National Military Park. The Daughters of Charity and the Battle of Gettysburg. Blog. August 22, 2019. https://npsgnmp.wordpress.com/category/hospitals/sisters-of-charity.
16. Holy Father Paul VI. Canonization of Elisabeth Ann Seton. Homily. September 14, 1975. https://www.vatican.va/content/paul-vi/en/homilies/1975/documents/hf_p-vi_hom_19750914.html.

Chapter 4: The Hierarchy and the Rules

1. Pope Paul VI. *Humanae Vitae*. Encyclical Letter. July 25, 1968. https://www.vatican.va/content/paul-vi/en/encyclicals/documents/hf_p-vi_enc_25071968_humanae-vitae.html.
2. Kauffman CJ. *Ministry and Meaning: A Religious History of Catholic Health Care in the United States*. New York: Herder and Herder, 1995.
3. Curran CE. *Diverse Voices in Modern US Moral Theology*. Washington, DC: Georgetown University Press, 2019.

4. Guttmacher Institute. Guttmacher Statistic on Catholic Women's Contraceptive Use. Policy Analysis. Guttmacher Institute. February 15, 2012. https://www.guttmacher.org/article/2012/02/guttmacher-statistic-catholic-womens-contraceptive-use.
5. Keenan JF. What Is Pope Francis' Effect on Healthcare? *America: The Jesuit Review*. May 18, 2018. https://www.americamagazine.org/politics-society/2018/05/18/what-pope-francis-effect-health-care.
6. Kaveny C. Pope Francis and Catholic Healthcare Ethics. *Theological Studies*. 2019; 80(1):186–201.
7. Salzman TA, Lawler MG. *Pope Francis and the Transformation of Health Care Ethics*. Washington, DC: Georgetown University Press, 2021.
8. Pope Francis. *Amoris Laetitia*. Post-Synodal Apostolic Exhortation. March 19, 2016. https://www.vatican.va/content/francesco/en/apost_exhortations/documents/papa-francesco_esortazione-ap_20160319_amoris-laetitia.html.
9. Pope Leo XIII. *Rerum Novarum*. Encyclical on Capitol and Labor. May 15, 1891. https://www.vatican.va/content/leo-xiii/en/encyclicals/documents/hf_l-xiii_enc_15051891_rerum-novarum.html.
10. DeBerri EP, Hug JE, Henriot PJ, Schultheis MJ. *Catholic Social Teaching: Our Best Kept Secret*. Maryknoll, NY: Orbis Books, 1992.
11. Lanari B. Seven Principles of Catholic Social Doctrine. *Homiletic and Pastoral Review*. 2009;110(3):52–57.
12. American Catholic Bishops. *Health and Health Care. A Pastoral Letter of the American Bishops*. November 19, 1981. (©USCCB, Washington, DC. All rights reserved. Used by permission.) https://www.usccb.org/issues-and-action/human-life-and-dignity/health-care/upload/health-and-health-care-pastoral-letter-pdf-09-01-43.pdf.
13. United States Catholic Bishops. *Economic Justice for All: Pastoral Letter on Catholic Social Teaching and the U.S. Economy*. (copyright USCCB, Washington, DC. All rights reserved. Used by permission.) Washington, DC: United States Catholic Bishops, 1986.
14. Catholic Church. *Catechism of the Catholic Church*. Liguori, MO; Liguori Publications, 1994.
15. Pope John Paul II. *Christifidelis Laici*. Post-Synodal Apostolic Exhortation. December 30, 1988. https://www.vatican.va/content/john-paul-ii/en/apost_exhortations/documents/hf_jp-ii_exh_30121988_christifideles-laici.html.
16. Gomes R. Pope on Synod: The Participation of Everyone, Guided by the Holy Spirit. *Vatican News*. October 9, 2021. https://www.vaticannews.va/en/pope/news/2021-10/pope-francis-discourse-moment-reflection-eve-inauguration-synod.html
17. Catholic Physicians' Guild. Ethical and Religious Directives for Catholic Hospitals. *The Linacre Quarterly*. 1948;15(3).
18. United States Conference of Catholic Bishops. *Ethical and Religious Directives for Catholic Health Care Services, Fifth Ed*. Washington, DC: United States Conference of Catholic Bishops, 2009.

19. United States Conference of Catholic Bishops: *Ethical and Religious Directives for Catholic Health Care Services, Sixth Ed.* Washington, DC: United States Conference of Catholic Bishops, 2018.
20. O'Rourke KD, Kofensteiner T, Hamel R. A Summary of the Development of the Ethical and Religious Directives for Catholic Health Care Services. *Health Progress.* November-December 2001. https://www.chausa.org/publications/health-progress/article/november-december-2001/a-brief-history#top.
21. Hamil R. The Ethical and Religious Directives: Looking Back to Move Forward. *Health Progress.* November-December 2019. https://www.chausa.org/docs/default-source/health-progress/100th-anniversary---the-ethical-and-religious-directives.pdf.
22. Penan H, Chen A. The Ethical & Religious Directives: What the 2018 Update Means for Catholic Hospital Mergers. *National Health Law Program.* January 2, 2019. https://healthlaw.org/resource/the-ethical-religious-directives-what-the-2018-update-means-for-catholic-hospital-mergers.
23. McCormick RA. Not What Catholic Hospitals Ordered. *The Linacre Quarterly.* 1972;39(1):7.
24. United States Conference of Catholic Bishops. *Doctrinal Note on the Moral Limits to Technological Manipulation of the Human Body.* March 20, 2023. https://www.usccb.org/resources/doctrinal-note-moral-limits-technological-manipulation-human-body
25. Boorstein M. U.S. Catholic Bishops to Create First Guidelines for Transgender Health Care. *The Washington Post.* June 16, 2023. https://www.washingtonpost.com/religion/2023/06/16/catholic-bishops-trans-health.
26. Congregation for the Doctrine of the Faith. *Samaritanus Bonus.* Letter. July 14, 2020. https://press.vatican.va/content/salastampa/en/bollettino/pubblico/2020/09/22/200922a.html.
27. Dignity Health. Important Information About Transgender Health Care at Dignity Health. Dignity Health website. https://www.dignityhealth.org/lgbtqcare/oursupport/transgender-health-care.
28. Shapiro N. Catholic Health Care Restrictions Lead WA Legislature to Eye Changes. *Seattle Times.* February 6, 2023. https://www.seattletimes.com/seattle-news/health/religious-health-care-restrictions-prompt-call-for-wa-merger-oversight.
29. Keenan JF. What Is Pope Francis' Effect on Health Care? *America: The Jesuit Review.* May 18, 2018. https://www.americamagazine.org/politics-society/2018/05/18/what-pope-francis-effect-health-care.

Chapter 5: The Impact of the Rules on Patient Care

1. Solomon T, Uttley L, HasBrouck P, Jung Y. *Bigger and Bigger: The Growth of Catholic Health Systems.* Community Catalyst. February 8, 2020. https://communitycatalyst.org/resource/bigger-and-bigger-the-growth-of-catholic-health-systems.
2. American Hospital Association. Hospital Operational and Demographic Data: FY 2020 AHA Annual Survey Database. Chicago: American Hospital Association. www.ahadata.com.

3. Rural Health Information Hub. Rural Hospitals. February 10, 2022. https://www.ruralhealthinfo.org.
4. Largest Healthcare Systems. *Modern Healthcare*. December 20, 2021; reissued with correction March 7, 2022.
5. Pew Research Center. Religious Landscape Study: Catholics. Pew Research Center. https://www.pewresearch.org/religion/religious-landscape-study/religious-tradition/catholic.
6. Drake C, Jarlenski M, Zhang Y, Polsky D. Market Share of US Catholic Hospitals and Associated Geographic Network Access To Reproductive Health Services. *JAMA Network Open*. 2020;3(1): e1920053–e1920053.
7. Cartwright AF, Bullington BW, Arora KS, Swartz JJ. Prevalence and County-Level Distribution of Births in Catholic Hospitals in the US in 2020. *JAMA*. 2023;329(11):937–939.
8. Hamilton BE, Martin JA, Osterman MJK. Births: Provisional Data for 2020. *Vital Statistics Rapid Release*. Report No. 012. National Center for Health Statistics. May 2021. https://www.cdc.gov/nchs/data/vsrr/vsrr012-508.pdf.
9. Daniels K, Abma JC. Current Contraceptive Status Among Women Aged 15–49: United States, 2015–2017. *NCHS Data Brief* No. 327. Centers for Disease Control and Prevention. December 2018. https://www.cdc.gov/nchs/data/databriefs/db327-h.pdf.
10. Jones RK. People of All Religions Use Birth Control and Have Abortions. Guttmacher Institute. October 19, 2020. https://www.guttmacher.org/article/2020/10/people-all-religions-use-birth-control-and-have-abortions.
11. Kaye J, Amiri B, Melling L, Dalven J. *Health Care Denied: Patients and Physicians Speak Out About Catholic Hospitals and the Threat to Women's Health and Lives*. New York: American Civil Liberties Union, May 2016. https://www.aclu.org/report/report-health-care-denied?redirect=report/health-care-denied.
12. Katz A. Letter for Mrs. Versailles. Center for Reproductive Rights. March 4, 2016. http://reproductiverights.org/wp-content/uploads/2018/10/CO-Versailles-Demand-Letter-FINAL.pdf.
13. Brown J. Another Colorado Hospital Stops Letting Women Get Their Tubes Tied, Renewing Questions About Reproductive Rights. *The Colorado Sun*. January 31, 2023.
14. Brown J. Colorado Hospitals That Won't Allow Women To Get Their Tubes Tied, Provide Gender-Affirming Care Will Have To Say So Publicly. *The Colorado Sun*. May 3, 2023. https://coloradosun.com/2023/05/03/colorado-hospitals-tubes-tied-transgender-health-public.
15. Guiahi M. Religious Refusals to Long-Acting Reversible Contraceptives in Catholic Settings: A Call for Evidence. *American Journal of Obstetrics and Gynecology*. 2020;222(4):S869-e1.
16. Shepherd K, Platt ER, Franke K, Boylan E. Bearing Faith: The Limits of Catholic Health Care for Women of Color. Law, Rights & Religion Project. Columbia Law School. January 2018. https://lawrightsreligion.law.columbia.edu/bearingfaith.

17. Medicaid and CHIP Payment and Access Commission (MACPAC). 2020. Chapter 5: Medicaid's Role in Maternal Health. In *June 2020 Report to Congress on Medicaid and CHIP*. Washington, DC: MACPAC, June 2020.
18. Sonfield A. A Fragmented System: Ensuring Comprehensive Contraceptive Coverage in All U.S. Health Insurance Plans. *Guttmacher Policy Review.* 2021;24:1–7.
19. Wilson CH, Lazorwitz A, Hyer J, Guiahi M. Concordance of Desired and Administered Postpartum Contraceptives among Emergency and Full Scope Medicaid Patients. *Women's Health Issues.* 2022;32(4):243–351.
20. Thomson-DeVeaux A, Barry-Jester AM. Insurers Can Send Patients To Religious Hospitals That Restrict Reproductive Care. *FiveThirtyEight.* August 1, 2018. https:// fivethirtyeight.com/features/how-insurers-can-send-patients-to-religious-hospitals-that-restrict-reproductive-care.
21. Gieseker R, Garcia-Ricketts S, Hasselbacher L, Stulberg D. Family Planning Service Provision in Illinois Religious Hospitals: Racial/Ethnic Variation in Access To Non-Religious Hospitals for Publicly Insured Women. *Contraception.* 2019;100(4):296–298.
22. Kramer RD, Higgins JA, Burns ME, Freedman LR, Stulberg D. Prevalence and Experiences of Wisconsin Women Turned Away From Catholic Settings Without Receiving Reproductive Care. *Contraception.* 2021:104(4):377–382.
23. Guiahi M, Teal SB, Swartz M, Huynh S, Schiller G, Sheeder J. What Are Women Told When Requesting Family Planning Services at Clinics Associated with Catholic Hospitals? A Mystery Caller Study. *Perspectives on Sexual and Reproductive Health.* 2017;49(4):207–212.
24. Hapenney S. Divergent Practices Among Catholic Hospitals in Provision of Direct Sterilization. *The Linacre Quarterly.* 2013:80(1):32–38.
25. Hill EL, Slusky DJG, Ginther DK. Reproductive Health Care in Catholic-owned Hospitals. *Journal of Health Economics.* 2019;65:48–62.
26. Smugar SS, Spina BJ, Merz JF. Informed Consent for Emergency Contraception: Variability in Hospital Care of Rape Victims. *American Journal of Public Health.* 2000;90(9):1372.
27. Federal Bureau of Investigation. FBI Crime in the United States 2018. FBI website. https://ucr.fbi.gov/crime-in-the-u.s/2018/crime-in-the-u.s.-2018/topic-pages/rape.
28. Centers for Disease Control and Prevention. *Youth Risk Behavior Survey Data Summary & Trends Report. 2011–2021.* CDC. https://www.cdc.gov/healthyyouth/data/yrbs/pdf/YRBS_Data-Summary-Trends_Report2023_508.pdf.
29. United States Conference of Catholic Bishops: *Ethical and Religious Directives for Catholic Health Care Services, Sixth Ed.* Washington, DC, 2018.
30. United States Supreme Court. *Dobbs, State Health Officer of the Mississippi Department of Health et al. v. Jackson Women's Health Organization et al.* Argued December 1, 2021—Decided June 24, 2022.
31. Nash E, Guarnieri I. Six Months Post-Roe, 24 US States Have Banned Abortion or Are Likely to Do So: A Roundup. Guttmacher Institute. January 2023.

https://www.guttmacher.org/2023/01/six-months-post-roe-24-us-states-have-banned-abortion-or-are-likely-do-so-roundup.
32. Zablocki A, Sutrina, MT. The Impact of State Laws Criminalizing Abortion. LexisNexis. September 27, 2022. https://www.lexisnexis.com/community/insights/legal/practical-guidance-journal/b/pa/posts/the-impact-of-state-laws-criminalizing-abortion.
33. Jones RK, Nash E, Cross L, Philbin J, Kristein M. Medication Abortion Now Accounts for More Than Half of All US Abortions. Guttmacher Institute. February 2022. https://www.guttmacher.org/article/2022/02/medication-abortion-now-accounts-more-half-all-us-abortions.
34. Chen DW, Belluck P. Wyoming Becomes First State to Outlaw the Use of Pills for Abortion. *The New York Times*. March 17, 2023.
35. Sparks G, Schumacher S, Presiado M, Kirzinger A, Brodie M. KFF Health Tracking Poll: Early 2023 Update On Public Awareness On Abortion and Emergency Contraception. Kaiser Family Foundation. February 1, 2023. https://www.kff.org/womens-health-policy/poll-finding/kff-health-tracking-poll-early-2023.
36. State Funding of Abortion Under Medicaid. Guttmacher Institute. June 1, 2023. https://www.guttmacher.org/state-policy/explore/state-funding-abortion-under-medicaid.
37. AP-NORC Center for Public Affairs Research. Most Catholic Americans Disagree with Hardline Positions of Church Leadership. June 2022. https://apnorc.org/projects/most-catholic-americans-disagree-with-hardline-positions-of-church-leadership.
38. Saad L. Pro-Choice' Identification Rises to Near Record High in U.S. GALLUP. June 2, 2022. https://news.gallup.com/poll/393104/pro-choice-identification-rises-near-record-high.aspx.
39. Neill S. Management of Early Pregnancy Loss. *JAMA*. 2023;329(16): 1399–1400.
40. American College of Obstetricians and Gynecologists. Early Pregnancy Loss FAQs. ACOG website. January 2022. https://www.acog.org/womens-health/faqs/early-pregnancy-loss.
41. Littlefield A. Abandoned: Stories of Catholic Healthcare Refusals. *Conscience Magazine*. November 4, 2020. https://www.catholicsforchoice.org/resource-library/abandoned-stories-of-catholic-healthcare-refusals.
42. Panelli DM, Phillips CH, Brady PC. Incidence, Diagnosis and Management of Tubal and Nontubal Ectopic Pregnancies: A Review. *Fertility Research and Practice*. 2015;1(1):1–20.
43. Condic ML, Harrison D. Treatment of an Ectopic Pregnancy: An Ethical Reanalysis. *The Linacre Quarterly*. 2018;85(3):241–251.
44. McIntyre A. Doctrine of Double Effect. In: Zalta EN (ed.) *The Stanford Encyclopedia of Philosophy*. Stanford, CA: Stanford University, 2006.
45. Frederiksen B, Ranji U, Gomez I, Salganicoff A. A National Survey of OBGYNs' Experiences After Dobbs. Kaiser Family Foundation. June 21, 2023. https://www.kff.org/womens-health-policy/report/a-national-survey-of-obgyns-experiences-after-dobbs.

46. Christian NT, Borges VF. What Dobbs Means for Patients with Breast Cancer. *New England Journal of Medicine.* 2022;387(9):765–776.
47. Borrero S, Talabi MB, Dehlendorf C. Confronting the Medical Community's Complicity in Marginalizing Abortion Care. *JAMA.* 2022;328(17):1701–1702.
48. National Institutes of Health. How Common Is Infertility? National Institute of Child Health and Human Development. February 8, 2018. https://www.nichd.nih.gov/health/topics/infertility/conditioninfo/common.
49. Read AP, Donnai D. What Can Be Offered to Couples at (Possibly) Increased Genetic Risk? *Journal of Community Genetics.* 2012;3:167–174.
50. NCBC Ethicists. Brief Statement on Transgenderism. The National Catholic Bioethics Center. February 22, 2017. https://www.ncbcenter.org/resources-and-statements-cms/brief-statement-on-transgenderism.
51. Di Camillo JA. Gender Transitioning and Catholic Health Care. *The National Catholic Bioethics Quarterly.* 2017;17(2):213–223.
52. Human Rights Campaign. Health Care Equity Index. Human Rights Campaign. https://www.hrc.org/resources/healthcare-equality-index.
53. United States Conference of Catholic Bishops Committee on Doctrine. Doctrinal Note on the Moral Limits to Technological Manipulation of the Human Body. United States Conference of Catholic Bishops. March 20, 2023.
54. Boorstein M. U.S. Catholic Bishops to Create First Guidelines for Transgender Health Care. *The Washington Post.* June 16, 2023. https://www.washingtonpost.com/religion/2023/06/16/catholic-bishops-trans-health.
55. Dignity Health. Important Information About Transgender Health Care at Dignity Health. Dignity Health website. https://www.dignityhealth.org/lgbtqcare/oursupport/transgender-health-care.
56. Hichborn M. *CommonSpirit Health and the Sex-Change Industry.* Lepanto Institute. May 2023.
57. Jenkins J. Catholic Nuns' Letter Declares Trans People 'Beloved and Cherished by God.' *Religious News Service.* March 31, 2023. https://religionnews.com/2023/03/31/letter-representing-thousands-of-catholic-nuns-declares-trans-people-beloved-and-cherished-by-god.
58. Shine R. Sisters of Mercy to Transgender Community: "We See You. . .We Love You! New Ways Ministry. May 13, 2023. https://www.newwaysministry.org/2023/05/13/sisters-of-mercy-to-transgender-community-we-see-you-we-love-you-and-more-news.
59. Collins SK. Critics Say US Bishops' New Statement on Transgender Health Care Lacks Sound Science and Trans Voices. *National Catholic Reporter.* March 21, 2023. https://www.ncronline.org/news/critics-say-us-bishops-new-statement-transgender-health-care-lacks-sound-science-and-trans.
60. Kohlhaas J. Transgender Healthcare and the Catholic Moral Vision. *New Ways Ministry.* April 10, 2023. https://www.newwaysministry.org/2023/04/10/transgender-healthcare-and-the-catholic-moral-vision.
61. Reed B. Pope Francis Calls for End to Anti-Gay Laws and LGBTQ+ Welcome from Church. *The Guardian.* January 25, 2023. https://www.theguardian.com/world/2023/jan/25/pope-francis-calls-for-end-to-anti-gay-laws-and-lgbtq-welcome.

62. Winfield N. Vatican Document Highlights Need for Concrete Steps for Women, 'Radical Inclusion' of LGBTQ+. *AP News.* June 20, 2023. https://apnews.com/article/vatican-synod-women-lgbtq-pope-abuse-63b13399c4cd363a7a086c7b513e6283.
63. Smith WJ. Catholic Hospital Can Be Sued for Refusing Transgender Hysterectomy. *National Review.* September 19, 2019.
64. Smith WJ. Maryland Catholic Hospital Liable for Refusing Transgender Hysterectomy. *National Review.* January 12, 2023.
65. Gomez I, Ranji U, Salganicoff A, Dawson L, Rosenzweig C, Kellenberg R, Gifford, K. Updates on Medicaid Coverage of Gender-Affirming Health Services. Kaiser Family Foundation. October 11, 2022. https://www.kff.org/womens-health-policy/issue-brief/update-on-medicaid-coverage-of-gender-affirming-health-services.
66. Alfonseca K. Map: Where Gender-affirming Care Is Being Targeted in the US. ABC News. April 10, 2023. https://abcnews.go.com/US/map-gender-affirming-care-targeted-us/story?id=97443087.
67. Institute of Medicine. *Approaching Death: Improving Care at the End of Life.* Washington, DC: The National Academies Press, 1997. https://doi.org/10.17226/5801.
68. Xu J, Murphy SL, Kochanek KD, Arias E. Mortality in the United States, 2018. *NCHS Data Brief, no 355.* Hyattsville, MD: National Center for Health Statistics, 2020. https://www.cdc.gov/nchs/data/databriefs/db355-h.pdf.
69. Cross SH, Warraich HJ. Changes in the Place of Death in the United States. *New England Journal of Medicine.* 2019;381(24):2369–2370.
70. Arias E, Tejada-Vera B, Ahmad F, Kochanek, K. Provisional Life Expectancy Estimates for 2020." *Vital Statistics Rapid Release.* Report No. 015. Centers for Disease Control and Prevention. July 2021. https://www.cdc.gov/nchs/data/vsrr/vsrr015-508.pdf.
71. Congregation for the Doctrine of the Faith. *Samaritanus Bonus.* Letter. July 14, 2020. https://press.vatican.va/content/salastampa/en/bollettino/pubblico/2020/09/22/200922a.html.
72. Truog RD. The Uncertain Future of the Determination of Brain Death. *JAMA.* 2023;329(12): 971–972.
73. Compassion and Choices. Our State Advocacy. Compassion and Choices website. https://www.compassionandchoices.org/state-advocacy.
74. Karlik M. Jury to Decide Whether Centura Improperly Fired Doctor Who Supported Aid-In-Dying, Appeals Court Rules. *Colorado Politics.* April 14, 2023. https://www.coloradopolitics.com/courts/jury-to-decide-whether-centura-properly-fired-doctor-who-supported-aid-in-dying/article_6632cd2c-db0c-11ed-93bf-a726c002bdef.html.
75. Wynia M. Colorado End-of-Life Options Act: A Clash of Organizational and Individual Conscience. *JAMA.* 2019;322 (20):1953–1954.
76. Hafner K. As Catholic Hospitals Expand, So Do Limits on Some Procedures. *The New York Times.* August 10, 2018. https://www.nytimes.com/2018/08/10/health/catholic-hospitals-procedures.html.

77. Meyer H. Most Catholic Hospitals Don't Disclose Religious Care Restrictions. *Modern Healthcare*. March 15, 2019.
78. Takahashi J, Cher A, Sheeder J, Teal S, Guiahi M. Disclosure of Religious Identity and Health Care Practices on Catholic Hospital Websites. *JAMA*. 2019;321(11):1103–1104.
79. Guiahi M, Helbin PE, Teal SB, Stulberg D, Sheeder J. Patient Views on Religious Institutional Health Care. *JAMA Network Open*. 2019;2(12):e1917008–e1917008.
80. Stulberg DB, Guiahi M, Hebert LE, Freedman LR. Women's Expectation of Receiving Reproductive Health Care at Catholic And Non-Catholic Hospitals. *Perspectives on Sexual and Reproductive Health*. 2019;51(3):135–142.
81. Guiahi M, Sheeder J, Stulberg D. Patient Perceptions of Healthcare Differences within Catholic Facilities. *American Journal of Obstetrics & Gynecology*. 2021;224(1):110–111.
82. Rouner J. St. Luke Asserts "Pro-Life" Stance in Conflicting New Patient Form. *Houston Press*. June 13, 2022. https://www.houstonpress.com/houston/Print?oid=13544174.
83. Colorado House Bill 23–1218. https://leg.colorado.gov/sites/default/files/2023a_1218_signed.pdf.

Chapter 6: Fulfilling Oaths and Following Conscience

1. American Hospital Association. *Hospital Operational and Demographic Data: FY 2020 AHA Annual Survey Database*. Chicago: American Hospital Association. www.ahadata.com.
2. Accreditation Council for Graduate Medical Education (ACGME). https://www.acgme.org.
3. Guiahi M, Hoover J, Swartz M, Teal S. Impact of Catholic Hospital Affiliation During Obstetrics and Gynecology Residency on the Provision of Family Planning. *Journal of Graduate Medical Education*. 2017;9(4):440–446.
4. Greek Medicine-Hippocratic Oath. National Library of Medicine. https://www.nlm.nih.gov/hmd/greek/greek_oath.html.
5. Oath of Maimonides. Dalhousie University Libraries. https://dal.ca.libguides.com.
6. American Medical Association. History of the Code. AMA website. https://www.ama-assn.org/sites/ama-assn.org/files/corp/media-browser/public/ethics/ama-code-ethics-history.pdf.
7. American Medical Association. Code of Medical Ethics. AMA website. (Used with permission of the American Medical Association. ©American Medical Association 2023. All rights reserved.) https://code-medical-ethics.ama-assn.org.
8. Stahl RY, Emanuel EJ. Physicians, Not Conscripts—Conscientious Objection in Health Care. *New England Journal of Medicine*. 2017;376(14):1380–1385.
9. The American College of Obstetricians and Gynecologists. The Limits of Conscientious Refusal in Reproductive Medicine. Committee Opinion Number 385. November 2007. https://www.acog.org/clinical/clinical-guidance/

committee-opinion/articles/2007/11/the-limits-of-conscientious-refusal-in-reproductive-medicine.

10. Curlin FA, Lawrence RE, Chin MH, Lantos JE. Religion, Conscience, and Controversial Clinical Practices. *New England Journal of Medicine.* 2007;356(6):593–600.

11. United States Conference of Catholic Bishops. *Ethical and Religious Directives for Catholic Health Care Services, Sixth Ed.* Washington, DC: United States Conference of Catholic Bishops, 2018.

12. Young A, Chaudhry HJ, Pei X, Arnhart K, Dugan M, Simons KB. FSMB Census of Licensed Physicians in the United States, 2020. *Journal of Medical Regulation.* 2021;107(2):57–64.

13. Stulberg DB, Hoffman Y, Dahlquist IH, Freedman LR. Tubal Ligation in Catholic Hospitals: A Qualitative Study of Ob–Gyns' Experiences. *Contraception.* 2014;90(4):422–428.

14. Ascension Wisconsin NE. Medical Staff Bylaws. https://healthcare.ascension.org/-/media/project/ascension/healthcare/legacy/markets/wisconsin/affinity-med-staff-services/amg-bylaws.pdf.

15. Derse AR. Fundamentals of Health Law: The Physician–Patient Relationship. *New England Journal of Medicine.* 2022;387(11):669–672.

16. Wynia MK. Professional Civil Disobedience — Medical-Society Responsibilities After Dobbs. *New England Journal of Medicine.* 2022;387(11):959–961.

17. Reingold RB, Gostin LO, Goodwin MB. Legal Risks and Ethical Dilemmas for Clinicians in the Aftermath of Dobbs. *JAMA.* 2022;328(17):1695–1696.

18. Constitution of the United States. https://constitution.congress.gov/constitution.

19. International Network of Civil Liberties Organizations. *Drawing the Line: Tackling Tensions Between Religious Freedom and Equality.* International Network of Civil Liberties Organizations. Buenos Aires, Argentina: INCLO, September 2015.

20. Church Amendments, 42 U.S.C. § 300a-7. U.S. Department of Health and Human Services. https://www.hhs.gov/sites/default/files/ocr/civilrights/understanding/ConscienceProtect/42usc300a7.pdf.

21. National Research Service Award Act. Public Law 93–348. July 12, 1974. https://www.govinfo.gov/content/pkg/STATUTE-88/pdf/STATUTE-88-Pg342.pdf.

22. Religious Freedom Restoration Act of 1993 HR 1308. https://www.congress.gov/bill/103rd-congress/house-bill/1308.

23. Brief of Amici Curiae Senator Daniel Coats and Representative David Weldon in Support of Defendants — Appellants and Reversal. 19–4254(L), 20–31, 20–32, 20–41. In the United States Court of Appeals for the Second Circuit. https://www.regent.edu/app/uploads/2020/06/CA2-Amicus-of-Coats-Weldon-NY-v-HHS.pdf.

24. Dubow S. "A Constitutional Right Rendered Utterly Meaningless": Religious Exemptions and Reproductive Politics, 1973–2014. *Journal of Policy History.* 2015;27(1):1–35.

25. The Weldon Amendment: Interfering with Abortion Coverage and Care. Guttmacher Institute. July 2021. https://www.guttmacher.org/fact-sheet/weldon-amendment.
26. U.S. Department of Health Human Services. Fact Sheet. Final Conscience Regulation. Office for Civil Rights. May 2, 2019. https://www.hhs.gov/guidance/document/fact-sheet-final-conscience-regulation.
27. Gostin LO. The "Conscience" Rule: How Will It Affect Patients' Access To Health Services? *JAMA.* 2019;321(22):2152–2153.
28. Sepper E. Toppling the Ethical Balance — Health Care Refusal and the Trump Administration. *New England Journal of Medicine.* 2019;381(10):896–898.
29. Chavkin W, Abu-Odeh D, Clune-Taylor C, Dubow S, Ferber M, Meyer IH. Balancing Freedom of Conscience and Equitable Access. *American Journal of Public Health.* 2018;108(110):1487.
30. Johnson SH. Proposed Regulations Favor Providers' Conscience Rights over Patients' Rights. *Hastings Center Report* 48. 2018;4:3–4.
31. Sawicki NN. Disentangling Conscience Protections. *Hastings Center Report* 48. 2018:5:14–22.
32. Weixel N. Biden Administration Seeks to Rescind Trump-Era 'Conscience' Protections for Health Workers. *The Hill.* December 29, 2022. https://thehill.com/policy/healthcare/3792368-biden-administration-seeks-to-rescind-trump-era-conscience-protections-for-health-workers/.
33. Centers for Medicare & Medicaid Services. Emergency Medical Treatment & Labor Act (EMTALA). CMS.gov. https://www.cms.gov/regulations-and-guidance/legislation/emtala.
34. Centers for Medicare & Medicaid Services. Reinforcement of EMTALA Obligations Specific to Patients Who Are Pregnant or Are Experiencing Pregnancy Loss. Memo QSO-22-22-Hospitals. CMS.gov. July 11, 2022. https://www.cms.gov/medicareprovider-enrollment-and-certificationsurveycertificationgeninfopolicy-and-memos-states-and/reinforcement-emtala-obligations-specific-patients-who-are-pregnant-or-are-experiencing-pregnancy-0
35. Carbajal E. CMS Probes 2 Hospitals Over EMTALA Violations. *Becker's Hospital Review.* May 2, 2023. https://www.beckershospitalreview.com/legal-regulatory-issues/cms-probes-2-hospitals-over-emtala-violations.html.
36. Suran M. Treating Cancer in Pregnant Patients After *Roe v Wade* Overturned. *JAMA.* 2022;328(17):1674–1676.
37. MacDonald A, Gershengorn HB, Ashana DC. The Challenge Of Emergency Abortion Care Following the Dobbs Ruling. *JAMA.* 2022;328(17):1691–1692.

Chapter 7: The Landscape of Catholic Healthcare

1. Morrisey MA. Health Insurance in the United States. Chicago, IL: Health Administration Press, 2013.
2. Editorial. Hospital Survey and Construction Act. *New England Journal of Medicine.* 1946;235:498.
3. Chung AP, Gaynor M, Richards-Shubik S. Subsidies and Structure: The Lasting Impact of the Hill-Burton Program on the Hospital Industry. Working

Paper 22037. NBER Working Paper Series. National Bureau of Economic Research. February 2016. http://www.nber.org/papers/w22037.
4. Schulte EJ. The Catholic Health Care Facility: Its Identity, Ownership and Control." *Catholic Law.* 1974;20:328.
5. Schumann JH. A Bygone Era: When Bipartisanship Led To Health Care Transformation. Public Radio Tulsa. October 2, 2016. https://www.npr.org/sections/health-shots/2016/10/02/495775518/a-bygone-era-when-bipartisanship-led-to-health-care-transformation.
6. Center for Medicare Advocacy. Medicare Enrollment Numbers. June 29, 2023. https://medicareadvocacy.org/medicare-enrollment-numbers.
7. Centers for Medicare and Medicaid Services. February 2023 Medicaid & CHIP Enrollment Data Highlights. Medicaid.gov. https://www.medicaid.gov/medicaid/program-information/medicaid-and-chip-enrollment-data/report-highlights/index.html.
8. Centers for Medicare and Medicaid Services. NHE Fact Sheet. CMS.gov. https://www.cms.gov/Research-Statistics-Data-and-Systems/Statistics-Trends-and-Reports/NationalHealthExpendData/NHE-Fact-Sheet.
9. Coughlin TA, Liska D. The Medicaid Disproportionate Share Hospital Payment Program: Background and Issues. The Urban Institute. October 1997. https://www.urban.org/sites/default/files/publication/71236/307025-The-Medicaid-Disproportionate-Share-Hospital-Payment-Program.PDF.
10. Medicaid and CHIP Payment and Access Commission. Disproportionate Share Hospital Payments. MACPAC.gov. https://www.macpac.gov/subtopic/disproportionate-share-hospital-payments.
11. The Centers for Medicare and Medicaid Services. 2020 CMS-HCRIS Financial Data: The Centers for Medicare & Medicaid Services (CMS) Healthcare Cost Report Information System (HCRIS). https://www.cms.gov/data-research/statistics-trends-and-reports/cost-reports.
12. American Hospital Association. Hospital Operational and Demographic Data: *FY 2020 AHA Annual Survey Database.* Chicago: American Hospital Association. www.ahadata.com.
13. Medicaid and CHIP Payment and Access Commission. March 2021 Report to Congress on Medicaid and CHIP. Macpac. https://www.macpac.gov/publication/march-2021-report-to-congress-on-medicaid-and-chip.
14. HealthCare.gov. The Children's Health Insurance Program (CHIP). https://www.healthcare.gov/medicaid-chip/childrens-health-insurance-program.
15. U.S. Department of Health and Human Services. New Reports Show Record 35 Million People Enrolled in Coverage Related to the Affordable Care Act, with Historic 21 Million People Enrolled in Medicaid Expansion Coverage. https://www.hhs.gov/about/news/2022/04/29/new-reports-show-record-35-million-people-enrolled-in-coverage-related-to-the-affordable-care-act.html.
16. Lee A, Ruhter J, Peters C, De Lew N, Sommers BD. National Uninsured Rate Reaches All-Time Low in Early 2022. Issue Brief No. HP-2022–23. Office of the Assistant Secretary for Planning and Evaluation, U.S. Department of Health and Human Services. August 2022. https://aspe.hhs.gov/sites/default/

files/documents/f2dedbf8a4274ae7065674758959567f/Uninsured-Q1–2022-Data-Point-HP-2022–23.pdf.
17. Lown Institute. Lown Hospital Institute Hospitals Index. https://lowninstitute.org/projects/lown-institute-hospitals-index.
18. Rau J, Spola C. Some of America's Wealthiest Hospital Systems Ended Up Even Richer, Thanks to Federal Bailouts. *The Washington Post.* April 1, 2021. https://www.washingtonpost.com/us-policy/2021/04/01/hospital-systems-cares-act-bailout.
19. Schwartz K, Lopez E, Rae M, Neuman T. What We Know About Provider Consolidation. Kaiser Family Foundation. September 2, 2020. https://www.kff.org/health-costs/issue-brief/what-we-know-about-provider-consolidation.
20. Fulton BD, Arnold DR, King JS, Montague AD, Greaney TL, Scheffler RM. The Rise of Cross-Market Hospital Systems and their Market Power in the US: Study Examines the Increase in Cross-Market Hospitals Systems and Their Market Power in the US." *Health Affairs.* 2022;41(11):1652–1660.
21. Navathe AS, Connolly JE. Hospital Consolidation: The Rise of Geographically Distant Mergers. *JAMA.* 2023;329(18):1547–1548.
22. Solomon T, Uttley L, HasBrouck P, Jung Y. *Bigger and Bigger: The Growth of Catholic Health Systems.* Community Catalyst. February 8, 2020. https://communitycatalyst.org/resource/bigger-and-bigger-the-growth-of-catholic-health-systems.
23. Fialka JJ. *Sisters: Catholic Nuns and the Making of America.* New York: St. Martin's Press, 2003.
24. Rosengren J. Meet the Millennial Nuns. *America: The Jesuit Review.* November 18, 2021. https://www.americamagazine.org/faith/2021/11/18/millennial-nuns-catholic-vocations-241800.
25. Largest Healthcare Systems. By the Numbers. *Modern Healthcare.* December 20, 2021. (Corrected version March 7, 2022.)
26. United States Conference of Catholic Bishops: *Ethical and Religious Directives for Catholic Health Care Services, Sixth Ed.* Washington, DC: United States Conference of Catholic Bishops, 2018.
27. Lagasse J. Intermountain, SCL Health Complete Merger, Creating 33-Hospital System. *HealthCare Finance.* April 6, 2022. https://www.healthcarefinancenews.com/news/intermountain-scl-health-complete-merger-creating-33-hospital-system.
28. Gilmore J. *We Came North: Centennial Story of the Sisters of Charity of Leavenworth.* St. Meinrad, IN: Abbey Press, 1961.
29. Brinkman M. *Emerging Frontiers: Renewal in the Life of Women Religious Sisters of Charity of Leavenworth 1955–2005.* Mahwah, NJ: Paulist Press, 2008.
30. SCL Health. SCL History. SCL Health. https://www.sclhealth.org/about/history.
31. Buelt EL, Goldberg C. Canon Law and Civil Law Interface: Diocesan Corporations. *Catholic Law.* 1995;36:69.

32. St. Joseph's Hospital. About Us. St. Joseph's Hospital. https://www.sclhealth.org/locations/saint-joseph-hospital/about.
33. St. Mary's Hospital. About Us. St. Mary's Hospital. https://www.sclhealth.org/locations/st-marys-medical-center/about.
34. Bellandi D. Making an Exempla of It: Denver Merger Details Spelled Out; Deal to Close Dec. 31. *Modern Healthcare.* October 6, 1997. https://www.modernhealthcare.com/article/19971006/PREMIUM/710060301/making-an-exempla-of-it-denver-merger-details-spelled-out-deal-to-close-dec-31.
35. Staff. SCL Health System, Community First Foundation Agree to Governance Changes of Exempla Healthcare. *Becker's Hospital Review.* August 2, 2012. https://www.beckershospitalreview.com/hospital-transactions-and-valuation/scl-health-system-community-first-foundation-agree-to-governance-changes-of-exempla-healthcare.html.
36. Intermountain Healthcare. Who We Are. Intermountain Healthcare. https://intermountainhealthcare.org/about/who-we-are/fast-facts.
37. Intermountain Healthcare. About Us. Intermountain Healthcare. https://intermountainhealthcare.org/about.
38. SCL Health. https://www.sclhealth.org.
39. Platte Valley Medical Center. About Us. Platte Valley Medical Center. https://www.sclhealth.org/locations/platte-valley-medical-center/about.
40. CommonSpirit. https://www.commonspirit.org.
41. Catholic Health Initiatives. https://www.catholichealthinitiatives.org.
42. Centura Health. https://www.centura.org.
43. Kacik A. CommonSpirit Health, AdventHealth Break up Centura Health JV. *Modern Healthcare.* February 14, 2023. https://www.modernhealthcare.com/mergers-acquisition/commonspirit-health-adventhealth-joint-venture-centura-health.
44. Hudson C. CommonSpirit to Buy Five Hospitals Despite Challenging Operating Environment. *Modern Healthcare.* February 15, 2023. https://www.modernhealthcare.com/finance/commonspirit-steward-health-care-hospitals-utah-hca-healthcare-ftc-centura.
45. Dignity Health. https://www.dignityhealth.org.
46. St. Mary's Medical Center. https://www.dignityhealth.org/bayarea/locations/stmarys.
47. CHI Health. Creighton University Medical Center. https://www.chihealth.com/en/location-search/cumcuc.html.
48. Centura. Centura-St. Anthony Hospital. https://www.centura.org/location/st-anthony-hospital.
49. Virginia Mason Franciscan Health. https://www.vmfh.org.
50. Bannow T, Meyer H. CHI-Dignity Merger Cleared by Vatican. *Modern Healthcare.* October 16, 2018. https://www.modernhealthcare.com/article/20181016/NEWS/181019911/chi-dignity-merger-cleared-by-vatican.
51. Sciacca A. Despite Doctors' Concerns, University of California Renews Ties With Religious Affiliates. *KFF Health News.* January 12, 2023. https://

kffhealthnews.org/news/article/despite-doctors-concerns-university-of-california-renews-ties-with-religious-affiliates.
52. Providence. History of Mother Joseph Province. Providence. https://www.providence.org/about/providence-archives/history-online/history-of-mother-joseph-province.
53. Providence. https://www.providence.org.
54. Providence. Historical Timelines. Providence Archives. https://www.providence.org/about/providence-archives/history-online/historical-timelines.
55. Kutscher B. Providence Health & Services to Partner with Pacific Medical Centers. *Modern Healthcare*. February 2, 2014. https://www.modernhealthcare.com/article/20140203/NEWS/302039967/providence-health-services-to-partner-with-pacific-medical-centers.
56. Ascension. https://healthcare.ascension.org.
57. Alexian Brothers. Congregation of Alexian Brothers History. http://www.alexianbrothers.org/aboutus/congregation-of-alexian-brothers-history.
58. Trinity Health. https://www.trinity-health.org.
59. The Academy of the Holy Cross. Sisters of the Holy Cross. https://www.academyoftheholycross.org/faith-justice/sisters-of-the-holy-cross.
60. Muoio D. Trinity Health Logs $298M Operating Loss Along with Merger-Fueled Revenue Growth in H1 2023." *Fierce Healthcare*. March 7, 2023. https://www.fiercehealthcare.com/providers/trinity-health-logs-298m-operating-loss-merger-fueled-revenue-growth-h1-2023.
61. Holy Cross Health. Holy Cross Hospital—Silver Spring. https://www.holycrosshealth.org/location/holy-cross-hospital-silver-spring-2.
62. Trinity Health. Trinity Health Ann Arbor Hospital. https://www.trinityhealthmichigan.org/location/trinity-health-ann-arbor-hospital.
63. Bon Secours Mercy Health. https://bsmhealth.org.
64. Sisters of Bon Secours. https://bonsecours.us.
65. Mercy Health. About Us. Mercy Health. https://www.mercy.com/about-us/history.
66. SSM Health. https://www.ssmhealth.com.
67. Muoio D. CommonSpirit Health Weathers $1.85B Net Loss in Fiscal 2022, Eyes Dual Challenges of Staffing and Inflation." *Fierce Healthcare*. September 23, 2022. https://www.fiercehealthcare.com/providers/commonspirit-health-weathers-185b-net-loss-fiscal-2022-now-eyes-dual-challenges-staffing
68. Muoio D. Providence Ends 2022 with –8.8% Operating Margin, $6.1B Net Loss. *Fierce Healthcare*. March 10, 2023. https://www.fiercehealthcare.com/providers/providence-ends-2022-88-operating-margin-61b-net-loss.
69. Muoio D. "Ascension Health Closes 2022 with $1.8B loss, -3.1% Operating Margin." *Fierce Healthcare*. September 19, 2022. https://www.fiercehealthcare.com/providers/ascension-health-closes-2022-18b-loss-31-operating-margin.
70. Ellison A. Trinity Health Reports $1.4B Annual Loss. *Becker's Hospital Review*. October 3, 2022. https://www.beckershospitalreview.com/finance/trinity-health-reports-1-4b-annual-loss.html.

71. Hudson C. Bon Secours Mercy Health's 2022 Losses Exceed $1 Billion. *Modern Healthcare.* March 23, 2023. https://www.modernhealthcare.com/finance/bon-secours-mercy-health-losses-2022.
72. Thomas N. SSM Health Reports $484M Loss Amid Excess Costs, Investment Problems. *Becker's Hospital Review.* November 22, 2022.
73. Pennic F. Hospitals Enter 2023 Facing 'New Normal' of Financial Uncertainty. *HIT Consultant.* February 28, 2023. https://hitconsultant.net/?s=Hospitals+Enter+2023.

Chapter 8: Mission Fidelity

1. Ascension. https://healthcare.ascension.org.
2. Bon Secours Mercy Health. https://bsmhealth.org.
3. CommonSpirit. https://www.commonspirit.org.
4. Providence. https://www.providence.org.
5. SSM Health. https://www.ssmhealth.com.
6. Trinity Health. https://www.trinity-health.org.
7. Tolbert J, Drake P, Damico A. Key Facts about the Uninsured Population. Kaiser Family Foundation. December 19, 2022. https://www.kff.org/uninsured/issue-brief/key-facts-about-the-uninsured-population.
8. Collins SR, Haynes LA, Masitha R. The State of U.S. Health Insurance in 2022. *Commonwealth Fund.* September 29, 2022. https://www.commonwealthfund.org/publications/issue-briefs/2022/sep/state-us-health-insurance-2022-biennial-survey.
9. Rae M, Claxton G, Amin K, Wager E, Ortaliza J, Cox C. The Burden of Medical Debt in the United States. Peterson-KFF Health System Tracker. https://www.healthsystemtracker.org/brief/the-burden-of-medical-debt-in-the-united-states.
10. Levey NN. Hundreds of Hospitals Sue Patients or Threaten Their Credit, a KHN Investigation Finds. Does Yours?" *KFF Health News.* December 21, 2022. https://kffhealthnews.org/news/article/medical-debt-hospitals-sue-patients-threaten-credit-khn-investigation.
11. Washington State Office of the Attorney General. Following AG's Charity Care Lawsuit, St. Joseph Parent Company CHI Franciscan Will Provide Up to $25 Million in Restitution, Debt Relief, and Fees. News Release. April 19, 2019. https://www.atg.wa.gov/news/news-releases/following-ag-s-charity-care-lawsuit-st-joseph-parent-company-chi-franciscan-will.
12. Silver-Greenberg J, Thomas K. They Were Entitled to Free Care. Hospitals Hounded Them to Pay." *The New York Times.* September 24, 2022. https://www.nytimes.com/2022/09/24/business/nonprofit-hospitals-poor-patients.html.
13. Thomas K, Silver-Greenberg J. How a Hospital Chain Used a Poor Neighborhood to Turn Huge Profits. *The New York Times.* September 24, 2022. https://www.nytimes.com/2022/09/24/health/bon-secours-mercy-health-profit-poor-neighborhood.html.

14. Robbins R, Thomas K, Silver-Greenberg J. How a Sprawling Hospital Chain Ignited Its Own Staffing Crisis. *The New York Times.* December 15, 2022. https://www.nytimes.com/2022/12/15/business/hospital-staffing-ascension.html.
15. DiGiorgio AM. 340B: Good Intentions in Need of Reform." *Health Affairs Forefront.* February 1, 2023. https://www.healthaffairs.org/content/forefront/340b-good-intentions-need-reform.
16. O'Sullivan MC. *The Sisters of Bon Secours in the United States 1881–1981: A Century of Caring.* York, PA: The Maple Press Company, 1982.
17. Halleman S. Illinois Nurses File Class Action Lawsuit Against Ascension Over Wage Issues. *HealthcareDIVE.* February 27, 2023. https://www.healthcaredive.com/news/illinois-nurses-file-class-action-suit-against-ascension.
18. Kelly K. Nurses in Texas and Kansas Make History with a Massive Strike. *truthout.* June 28, 2023. https://truthout.org/articles/nurses-in-texas-and-kansas-make-history-with-a-massive-strike.
19. Solomon T, Uttley L, HasBrouck P, Jung Y. *Bigger and Bigger: The Growth of Catholic Health Systems.* Community Catalyst. February 8, 2020. https://communitycatalyst.org/resource/bigger-and-bigger-the-growth-of-catholic-health-systems
20. American Hospital Association. Hospital Operational and Demographic Data: *FY 2020 AHA Annual Survey Database.* Chicago: American Hospital Association. www.ahadata.com
21. Lown Hospital Index. https://lowninstitute.org/projects/lown-institute-hospitals-index
22. Godwin J, Levinson Z, Hulver S. The Estimated Value of Tax Exemption for Nonprofit Hospitals Was About $28 Billion in 2020." Kaiser Family Foundation. March 14, 2023. https://www.kff.org/health-costs/issue-brief/the-estimated-value-of-tax-exemption-for-nonprofit-hospitals-was-about-28-billion-in-2020.
23. Zare H, Gabow P. Influence of Not-for-Profit Hospital Ownership Type on Community Benefit and Charity Care. *Journal of Community Health.* 2023;48(2):199–209.
24. Healey M. The Attorney General's Community Benefits Guidelines for Non-Profit Hospitals. Mass.gov. February 2018. https://www.mass.gov/doc/updated-nonprofit-hospital-community-benefits-guidelines/download.
25. Bai G, Letchuman S, Hyman DA. Do Nonprofit Hospitals Deserve Their Tax Exemption? *The New England Journal of Medicine.* 2023;389(3):196–197.
26. Bai G, Zare H, Eisenberg MD, Polsky D, Anderson GF. Analysis Suggests Government and Nonprofit Hospitals' Charity Care Is Not Aligned With Their Favorable Tax Treatment. *Health Affairs.* 2021;40(4):629–636.
27. Lown Institute Hospital Index. Methodology. https://lownhospitalsindex.org/rankings/our-methodology.
28. Lown Institute. Fair Share Spending. https://lownhospitalsindex.org/2023-fair-share-spending.

29. Brubaker H. School District Scores Major Win over Tower Health in Property-Tax Cases. *Philadelphia Inquirer.* February 10, 2023.
30. Lown Institute. Hospital Community Benefit Policy Watch. https://lowninstitute.org/hospital-community-benefit-policy-watch.
31. DiDonato P. *Immigrant Saint: The Life of Mother Cabrini.* Auckland, NZ: Pickle Partners Publishing, 2017.
32. United States Conference of Catholic Bishops. *Ethical and Religious Directives for Catholic Health Care Services, Sixth Ed.* Washington DC: United States Conference of Catholic Bishops, 2018.
33. Largest Healthcare Systems. By the Numbers. *Modern Healthcare.* December 20, 2021; Corrected version March 7, 2022.
34. Cohrs R. How America's Largest Catholic Hospital System Is Moonlighting as a Private Equity Firm. *STAT.* November 16, 2021. https://www.statnews.com/2021/11/16/ascensioninvestigation-moonlighting-private-equity-firm.
35. Winters MS. Ascension Health Commits Structural Sins Of Income Inequality, Capitalist Excess. *National Catholic Reporter.* November 29, 2018. https://www.ncronline.org/opinion/distinctly-catholic/ascension-health-commits-structural-sins-income-inequality-capitalist.
36. Senator Baldwin Demands Answers from Ascension on Conflicting Priorities and Impact on Wisconsin Patients. Senator Tammy Baldwin Press Release. February 13, 2023. https://www.baldwin.senate.gov/news/press-releases/senator-baldwin-demands-answers-from-ascension-on-conflicting-priorities-and-impact-on-wisconsin-patients.
37. Salins MJ, Friedlander M. Update on Health Care Joint Venture Arrangements. US Internal Revenue Service. https://www.irs.gov/pub/irs-tege/eotopicd00.pdf.
38. CommonSpirit. 2022 Philanthropy Annual Report. CommonSpirit. https://www.gettoknowphilanthropy.info.
39. Murphy B. Ascension Rakes in Charitable Dollars. *Urban Milwaukee.* January 17, 2023. https://urbanmilwaukee.com/2023/01/17/murphys-law-ascension-rakes-in-charitable-dollars.
40. Providence Foundation. https://foundation.providence.org.
41. Bon Secours Mercy Health Foundation. Financial Information. https://givebsmh.org/bon-secours-mercy-health-foundation/about/financial-information.
42. Bon Secours Mercy Health Foundation. Nonprofit Explorer. *Pro Publica.* https://projects.propublica.org/nonprofits/organizations/201072726.
43. SSM Health Foundation. Nonprofit Explorer. *Pro Publica.* https://projects.propublica.org/nonprofits/organizations/874109859.
44. United States Catholic Bishops. *Economic Justice for All: Pastoral Letter on Catholic Social Teaching and the U.S. Economy.* Washington, DC: United States Catholic Bishops, 1986. (©USCCB, Washington, DC. All rights reserved. Used with permission.
45. Kaufman AC. Pope Francis: 'Inequality Is the Root of Social Evil.'" *HUFFPOST.* April 28, 2014. https://www.huffpost.com/entry/pope-francis-tweet-inequality_n_5227563.

46. Hudson C. The Latest Trends in Executive Compensation. *Modern Healthcare.* July 17, 2023.
47. Shrider EA, Kollar M, Chen F, Semega J. Income and Poverty in the United States: 2020. *United States Census Bureau.* September 14, 2021. https://www.census.gov/library/publications/2021/demo/p60-273.html.
48. ZipRecruiter. https://www.ziprecruiter.com/Salaries/Hospital-Housekeeper-Salary-per-Hour.
49. U.S. Bureau of Labor Statistics. Occupational Employment and Wage Statistics. 29-1141 Registered Nurses. May 2022. https://www.bls.gov/oes/current/oes291141.htm..
50. Leapfrog Group. Leapfrog Safety Grade Scoring Methodology. Fall 2022. https://www.hospitalsafetygrade.org/media/file/Safety-Grade-Methodology-Fall-20222.pdf.

www.ingramcontent.com/pod-product-compliance
Lightning Source LLC
Chambersburg PA
CBHW072237290426
44111CB00012B/2128

This is a passionate dissent against the financialization of Catholic healthcare institutions and the extension of church doctrine into realms where it does not belong. Gabow's voice, grounded in church teachings, needs to be heard — in statehouses, in Congress, in the Vatican, in C-suites, and by everyone who cares about the future of American healthcare.

Merrill Goozner
Former Editor and Columnist for *Modern Healthcare*
Editor and Publisher of GoozNews, an online healthcare newsletter

As a life-long Catholic, a doctor for 50 years, and the top administrator of a safety-net hospital for 20 years, Patricia Gabow is uniquely qualified to trace the development and identify the tensions between the Catholic Church and its hospitals.

After describing the roots of the Catholic commitment to health in scripture and the early Church, she traces the dramatic evolution of Catholic hospitals in the United States, from the singular commitment of women religious in caring for the sick, to the struggle of Church authorities to maintain the Catholic character of their institutions, to the acute challenges posed by the onset of the massive healthcare systems that are currently reshaping Catholic hospitals.

Dr. Gabow closes by charting a pathway for revitalizing the Catholic commitment to caring for the sick, especially the poor, thus rekindling the vision of the Church and its hospitals as the fruit of a marriage made in heaven.

Michael J. Baxter, PhD
Department of Religious/Catholic Studies
Regis University
Denver, Colorado

I thoroughly enjoyed this book! I learned, was challenged, and laughed — my criteria for a good read.

With careful referencing and inclusion of scripture, Dr. Gabow delineates the history, mission, and foundational role Catholic healthcare institutions played in caring for poor, vulnerable, and marginalized Americans. As financial and secular forces changed Catholic healthcare, Gabow examines the ways it strayed from its noble past and offers a framework for getting back on track. Gabow doesn't pull any punches. Students of US healthcare, especially those concerned with health equity, will find this a must read.

Risa Lavizzo-Mourey
President and CEO Emerita
Robert Wood Johnson Foundation

Endorsements for *The Catholic Church and Its Hospitals: A Marriage Made in Heaven?*

Like the nuns who trained her, Dr. Gabow has never taken no for an answer. She always seeks the yes that will lead to better medical care for those in need. When other cities shut down their safety-net hospitals, Dr. Gabow built hers up. After decades of leading the way in developing sustainable systems for caring for the indigent ill, she delivers an urgent plea that all policymakers, administrators, and clinicians should heed. All should attend to her trenchant call for an equitable version of Catholic healthcare.

Abraham Nussbaum, MD
Chief Education Officer, Denver Health
Professor of Psychiatry, University of Colorado School of Medicine
Author of Progress Notes: One Year In the Future of Medicine.

I couldn't put this book down. In her latest blockbuster, Dr. Gabow diligently traces the path that Catholic healthcare in America has followed, from its altruistic roots to its current role as a major player in the healthcare landscape. Her clarion call for transparency could not be more timely, as medical practice has achieved a level of sophistication that puts it more and more at theological and philosophical odds with basic tenets of Catholicism. It is an important conflict in need of resolution, and Dr. Gabow not only lays out the issues but proposes a path forward in this courageous work.

Nanette Santoro, MD
Professor and E. Stewart Taylor Chair of Obstetrics and Gynecology
University of Colorado School of Medicine

In one of the largest Catholic health systems where I served as vice president, we often said "no margin no mission" to justify our choices. As I connected with Dr. Patty Gabow, she mentioned writing this book. She may be the only person qualified to do so. She is a physician, a former CEO of the largest safety net healthcare systems in Colorado, a national leader in delivery system innovation and care for vulnerable populations, and a practicing Catholic. Dr. Gabow takes us on a journey from the very beginning of Catholic healthcare, through the many facets of care delivery today. She thoughtfully questions current practices and offers ideas for moving forward. May her work provide grounding for future discussions and actions that improve care for every American, especially the most vulnerable.

Evon Halladay, MBA
Former Vice President, Catholic Health Initiatives